NEW DRUGS
(2005 - 2009)
and
COMPARISON RATINGS

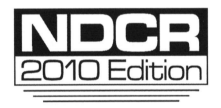

Daniel A. Hussar

Copyright © 2010 and published by Moore Road Press at King of Prussia, PA 19406. All rights reserved. None of the content of this publication may be reproduced, stored in a retrieval system, resold, redistributed, or transmitted in any form or by any means (electronic, mechanical, photocopying, recording, or otherwise) without the prior written permission of the publisher. *NDCR 2010* and *NDCR* are registered trademarks of Moore Road Press.

The product descriptions in *NDCR 2010* include all information made available by Daniel A. Hussar. The publisher does not warrant or guarantee any product, and does not perform any independent analysis of the information provided. Inclusion of a product in *NDCR 2010* does not represent an endorsement, and the publisher does not necessarily advocate the use of any product listed.

This edition of *NDCR 2010* contains the latest information available when the book went to press.

Table of Contents

Goals

The primary goals in the development of this book are to provide the most important information regarding the newest therapeutic agents marketed in the United States in an easy-to-use format, and to provide useful comparisons between the new drugs and other drugs already on the market that have related properties and/or uses.

The complexity of many of the new drugs often results in very lengthy product labeling (package inserts), as well as the availability of extensive additional information. This book is not intended to be an all-inclusive discussion of new drugs but, rather, is developed to provide the most important and practical information regarding these agents. When additional information is needed, more comprehensive references and/or the product labeling should be consulted.

About the Author

Daniel A. Hussar earned his B.S., M.S., and Ph.D. degrees in Pharmacy at the Philadelphia College of Pharmacy and Science, and is a licensed pharmacist in Pennsylvania. He holds the position of Remington Professor of Pharmacy at his alma mater (now the Philadelphia College of Pharmacy at the University of the Sciences in Philadelphia) where he has served on the full-time faculty since 1966. From 1975 to 1984 he served as Dean of Faculty at this institution. His faculty service has included the responsibility for teaching courses such as Pharmacy and Therapeutics, Nonprescription Drug Therapy, Pharmacy Ethics, Contemporary Issues in Pharmacy, Topics in Pharmacotherapeutics, and Dispensing Pharmacy, and as a participant in a team-taught Pharmacotherapeutics course sequence.

Dr. Hussar has written and spoken extensively on the topics of New Drugs, Drug Interactions, and Patient Compliance. His publications include coverage of all the new therapeutic agents that have been marketed in the United States during the last 40 years. His papers on New Drugs are published regularly in pharmacy and nursing journals and he speaks frequently on this topic to pharmacists, physicians, and nurses. He also has written numerous editorials regarding important issues facing the profession of pharmacy and the health care system. He currently serves as the Author/Editor of *The Pharmacist Activist*, a monthly newsletter, and has previously served as the Author/Editor of *The Drug Advisor*, and as Chief Pharmacy Editor of *Pharmacy Today*.

Dr. Hussar is a member of and active participant in numerous professional and civic organizations. He has served as President of the Drug Information Association and Pennsylvania Pharmaceutical Association, on the Board of Trustees of the American Pharmacists Association, and on the Board of Directors of World Vision. He currently serves on the Board of Directors of the Christian Pharmacists Fellowship International. The awards and recognitions he has received include the Distinguished Pharmacy Educator Award of the American Association of Colleges of Pharmacy, the Hugo Schaefer Award of the American Pharmacists Association, the Rho Chi Pharmacy Honor Society Lecture Award, and the Annual Alumni Award of the Philadelphia College of Pharmacy and Science.

Dr. Hussar and his wife Suzanne reside in Newtown Square, Pennsylvania. Their three sons, Eric with his wife Terra and sons Alex and Wesley and daughters Anna Kathryn and Cora, Christopher with his wife Carmen and daughter Pippa, and Timothy also reside in Pennsylvania.

Preface

I am privileged to have had numerous opportunities to write and speak on the topic of, "New Drugs." The questions I receive most often from pharmacists and other health professionals include:

"How does the new drug compare with the older drugs with which I am already familiar?"

"Does the new drug have advantages over the older drugs, or is it a 'me-too' drug?

To more effectively respond to these questions in an objective manner, I developed the New Drug Comparison Rating (NDCR) system in 2002 (see page xi). The response from health professionals who have used this system to assist in preliminarily determining the relative importance of a new drug has been very positive.

Objective information regarding the newest drugs is often not readily available. Although the product labeling for many of the individual agents may be quickly accessed on the Food and Drug Administration or pharmaceutical company websites, this information is not sufficient to permit a comparison with other medications having the same or similar uses. This book has been developed with a goal of providing content and a format that will facilitate timely user access to the most important and practical information regarding the 112 new therapeutic agents that have been marketed in the 2005-2009 period. The second goal is to identify older drugs to which a new drug is most similar in activity, the advantages and disadvantages of the new drug, and a rating that is a useful measure of the relative importance of the new drug. These features are unique with my coverage of new drugs in recent years, and this is the first comprehensive compilation of the information and ratings for the newest drugs, now in its second (2010) edition.

The development of this rating system and the format for providing this information is still a work in progress. I welcome your comments regarding its usefulness and your suggested revisions.

Daniel A. Hussar

Acknowledgments

I greatly value the professional motivation that I experience from the interaction with my students, faculty colleagues, and my former students and other pharmacists who are committed to patient care, the optimization of drug therapy, and the advancement of the profession of pharmacy. I greatly appreciate the encouragement from the many pharmacists who regularly attend my presentations on new drugs. Their commitment to learn about the newest drugs on a continuing basis is the reason for which I have extended and expanded my involvement with this topic.

The expertise, enthusiasm, and encouragement of Patrick Polli, Christopher Polli, and Jeff Zajac of NEWS-Line Publishing is very much appreciated. Although I developed the content, it is their expertise that has resulted in the production of a book.

My wife Sue, also a pharmacist, has been a continuing source of assistance, encouragement, and inspiration. On the occasions in which I was tempted to conclude that this project was too time-consuming to persist with it, it was her encouragement that prompted me to persevere.

Daniel A. Hussar

User Guide

Information is provided for the new <u>therapeutic</u> agents marketed in the 2005-2009 period. New diagnostic agents and products such as vaccines that have been developed to prevent disease are not included. Much of the information for each new drug is provided in outline form to facilitate rapid identification of specific information the user is seeking. The format used in providing information about the individual drugs is noted below with additional comments to designate the extent or limits of the information provided.

Generic name (Trade name – Manufacturer)   Therapeutic Class or Use

Year in which drug was first marketed: This may not always correspond to the year in which the drug was approved by the FDA. For example, a drug which the FDA approved late in a calendar year is often not actually marketed until the beginning of the next calendar year.

New Drug Comparison Rating (NDCR): This rating provides the author's assessment of the relative importance of the new drug when compared with other drugs to which it is most similar (see New Drug Comparison Rating system – page xi). The rating is determined at the time the drug is first marketed and is not subsequently changed (e.g., when a drug is approved for additional indications).

Indication: If the drug is not administered orally, the route of administration is designated first, followed by the specific indication(s). The indication(s) for most of the drugs is usually provided verbatim from the product labeling. Additional indications that have been approved since the drug was initially marketed are usually identified as "subsequently approved" to distinguish them from the initial indication(s) considered in the determination of the New Drug Comparison Rating.

Comparable drugs: The older drug(s) to which the new drug is most similar in properties and/or uses, and can best be compared, is(are) identified. In some situations, such as when a new drug is the first agent to be approved for a particular disorder, there are not any other drugs with which the new drug may be appropriately compared.

Advantages: Noteworthy advantages of the new drug, when compared with the older drug(s), are specifically identified.

Disadvantages: Noteworthy disadvantages or limitations of the new drug, when compared with the older drug(s), are specifically identified.

Most important risks/adverse events: The potential problems identified in this section include risks/adverse events that are typically identified in the product labeling as contraindications, warnings, precautions, risk during pregnancy, and potentially clinically important drug interactions.

Most common adverse events: The incidences noted for the adverse events are typically those reported in the clinical trials used in support of the New Drug Application submitted to the FDA, and that are identified in the product labeling. The adverse events identified are those that have been reported most frequently, and do not represent a complete listing of the adverse events experienced with the use of the drug.

Usual dosage: For many drugs, situations that warrant dosage adjustment are identified in addition to the usual dosage. However, the product labeling should be consulted for more specific dosage recommendations in circumstances in which a dosage other than the usual dosage would be considered.

Products: Many of the drugs that are administered parenterally have guidelines and/or restrictions regarding storage, constitution, dilution, and administration that go beyond the scope of coverage in this book. The product labeling should be consulted for more specific recommendations regarding the use of these products.

Comments: This section typically provides a description of the new drug, its mechanism of action, and its relationship to comparable drugs. A summary of the results of the clinical studies in which it was evaluated is often provided. When the drug has been approved for the treatment of a rare disorder, the condition is briefly described to provide a context for the role of the drug in treatment. Additional pertinent information that has not been provided earlier, or to expand on information provided in an earlier section, is provided for some drugs.

Although the New Drug Comparison Rating for a new drug is determined at the time it is initially marketed, and is not subsequently changed, the information for the new drugs has been updated to include pertinent information (e.g., new indications, warnings, formulations) that has become available since the time that it was first marketed. This information is typically identified in the pertinent section of the information for the drug and/or with a notation to see the Comments section for added information.

The first index facilitates access to the information for the new drugs based on their therapeutic classification and/or indication. Additional indications that have been approved since the new drugs were initially marketed are also included in this index. However, newer indications for drugs that were marketed before 2005 are not included. The second index facilitates access to the information for the new drugs based on their generic and trade names.

For almost all of the new drugs, there are no or few studies that have been published. Therefore, the product labeling as approved by the Food and Drug Administration is the source of much of the specific information provided for the new drugs. The author has identified the comparable drugs, advantages, and disadvantages, determined the New Drug Comparison Ratings, and provided the opinions included in the Comments section.

New Drug Comparison Rating (NDCR) System

The New Drug Comparison Rating (NDCR) system was developed for the purpose of providing a systematic approach in assessing the relative importance of a new drug. A rating from 1 to 5 (with 5 being the highest rating) is assigned for each new drug. The rating is based on a comparison of the new drug with related drugs already marketed, unless there are no other drugs to which the new agent can be appropriately compared. Specific advantages and disadvantages are identified and, with other pertinent information, are used as the basis for the determination of the rating. Thus, multiple parameters are evaluated in the determination of the numerical ratings which correspond to the overall opinions that are noted below:

> 5 = important advance (e.g., first drug approved for the indication)
> 4 = significant advantage(s) (e.g., with respect to use/effectiveness, safety, administration)
> 3 = no or minor advantage(s)/disadvantage(s), or advantage(s) and disadvantage(s) of similar importance
> 2 = significant disadvantage(s) (e.g., with respect to use/effectiveness, safety, administration)
> 1 = important disadvantage(s)

The development of a new drug that is the first drug to be approved for a particular clinical disorder is the most frequent reason for which the highest rating of 5 would be assigned, even if the drug would only be used in a small number of patients (e.g., as with an orphan drug). In some situations in which comparable drugs are already marketed, the advantages of the new drug are so important and clearly demonstrated that a rating of 5 has been assigned.

A rating of 4 is also a positive rating that reflects significant overall advantages for the new drug, even though the drug may have some significant disadvantages. In some situations, the advantages may warrant use of the new drug in preference to the comparable drugs identified. However, such a decision must be made individually for each drug, and the assignment of a rating of 4 must not be interpreted that the new drug should be considered the treatment of choice for the condition for which it has been approved. For example, most of the new antineoplastic and antiretroviral agents have been given a rating of 4 because of the importance of their advantage of being effective in some patients who are refractory/resistant to, or cannot tolerate, the usual treatment of first choice. Some of these drugs have indications for use only after the failure of prior therapies, but the importance of what may be their only advantage (that may result in a life-prolonging benefit) is considered to provide an overall advantage even if the drug has multiple less important disadvantages.

A rating of 3 is assigned to new drugs for which neither advantages nor disadvantages distinguish it from comparable drugs to an extent that would provide an overall rating that is positive (4 or 5) or negative (2 or 1). Examples include drugs that are sometimes referred to as "me-too" drugs. Some new drugs may have a significant advantage and a significant disadvantage but, if these differences are of generally similar importance, a rating of 3 would be assigned.

A rating of 2 is assigned to new drugs in which there are significant disadvantages and no or less important advantages. A rating of 1, representing important disadvantages, should be unexpected in view of the cost and effort expended by a pharmaceutical company to obtain approval for a new drug and bring it to market.

The New Drug Comparison Rating is determined at the time that a new drug is initially marketed and is not subsequently changed. However, the relative importance of a drug can change for a number of reasons (e.g., completion of additional studies that result in the approval of new indications, identification of additional risks, approval of newer comparable drugs that have significant advantages), and such changes are identified in the information provided for these drugs.

Studies in which a new drug is directly compared with a drug or drugs to which it is most similar would be of great value in determining the relative importance of a new drug and in determining a New Drug Comparison Rating. However, such studies are seldom conducted if the company developing the drug can obtain FDA approval based on placebo-controlled studies.

Although the cost of medications is a very important consideration with respect to their use, this has not been included in the determination of the New Drug Comparison Ratings, and the ratings are based on the properties, advantages, and disadvantages that pertain to the clinical use of the new drug and the comparable drugs.

Abatacept (Orencia – Bristol-Myers Squibb)
Antiarthritic Agent
2006

New Drug Comparison Rating (NDCR) = 4 (significant advantages)

Indications:

Administered via intravenous infusion for reducing signs and symptoms, inducing major clinical response, slowing the progression of structural damage, and improving physical function in adult patients with moderately to severely active rheumatoid arthritis who have had an inadequate response to one or more disease-modifying antirheumatic drugs (DMARDs) such as methotrexate or tumor necrosis factor (TNF) antagonists (e.g., etanercept [Enbrel]); may be used alone or concomitantly with DMARDs other than TNF antagonists. (subsequently revised to include "inhibiting [rather than slowing] the progression of structural damage" and to delete the restriction for use in patients "who have had an inadequate response to one or more disease-modifying drugs;" revisions also include the additional indication for reducing signs and symptoms in pediatric patients 6 years of age and older with moderately to severely active polyarticular juvenile idiopathic arthritis; may be used as monotherapy or concomitantly with methotrexate).

Comparable drugs:

Adalimumab (Humira), etanercept (Enbrel), infliximab (Remicade).

Advantages:

- Unique mechanism of action (inhibits the action of several mediators of inflammation).
- Is effective in some patients in whom there was an inadequate response with etanercept.
- Less frequent administration (compared with etanercept and adalimumab).

Disadvantages:

- Labeled indications are more limited.
- Not indicated for first-line use in patients with rheumatoid arthritis (indications have been subsequently revised to permit first-line use).
- Must be administered intravenously (compared with adalimumab and etanercept that are administered subcutaneously).
- Not indicated for pediatric use (compared with etanercept) (indications have been subsequently revised to include pediatric patients 6 years of age and older).

Most important risks/adverse events:

Infections (treatment should be discontinued if a patient develops a serious infection); should not be used concurrently with a TNF antagonist or anakinra (Kineret) because of a greater risk of infection; possible increased risk of malignancies; frequency of adverse events is higher in patients with chronic obstructive pulmonary disease; infusion-related reactions/hypersensitivity reactions; (additional risks/precautions include screening for latent tuberculosis infection prior to initiating therapy [patients testing positive should be treated prior to initiating abatacept]; avoiding the administration of live vaccines concurrently or within 3 months of discontinuation of treatment; possible blunting the effectiveness of some immunizations; immunizations for pediatric patients should be brought up to date prior to initiating treatment).

Most common adverse events:

Headache (18%), dizziness (9%), hypertension (7%), infections (5% to 13%) including upper respiratory tract infection, nasopharyngitis, sinusitis, urinary tract infection, influenza, and bronchitis.

Usual dosage:

Administered via intravenous infusion over 30 minutes; adults – 750 mg for patients weighing between 60 and 100 kg; 500 mg for patients weighing less than 60 kg; 1 gram for patients weighing more than 100 kg; following the administration of the first dose, the second and third doses should be administered 2 weeks and 4 weeks later, and subsequent doses every 4 weeks thereafter; (patients 6 to 17 years of age weighing less than 75 kg – 10 mg/kg at the intervals noted for adults).

Products:

Vials – 250 mg (should be stored in a refrigerator).

Comments:

Abatacept is a soluble fusion protein produced by recombinant DNA technology. It consists of the extracellular domain of the human cytotoxic T lymphocyte-associated antigen 4 (CTLA-4) linked to immunoglobulin G1 (IgG1). Designated as a selective costimulation modulator, abatacept inhibits T-cell (T lymphocyte) activation and has a unique combination of mechanisms of action compared to its predecessors. Abatacept inhibits the production of TNF-alpha, interferon-gamma, and interleukin-2. The studies in which abatacept was evaluated included patients who had been previously treated with methotrexate or etanercept but did not experience an adequate response with these agents. Abatacept was effective in some of these patients, thereby further extending the usefulness of this group of agents. Although the labeled indications for abatacept are much more limited than with the comparable drugs, its indications can be expected to expand as additional studies are completed.

As with the related drugs, patients treated with abatacept have a greater risk of infection and, possibly, malignancies. Although the overall frequencies of malignancy were similar in the abatacept- and placebo-treated patients, more cases of lung cancer were reported in patients treated with abatacept.

AbobotulinumtoxinA (Dysport – Ipsen)
Agent for Cervical Dystonia
2009

New Drug Comparison Rating (NDCR) = 3 (no or minor advantages/disadvantages)

Indications:
Administered intramuscularly for the treatment of adults with cervical dystonia to reduce the severity of abnormal head position and neck pain in both toxin-naïve and previously treated patients; also indicated for the temporary improvement in the appearance of moderate to severe glabellar lines associated with procerus and corrugator muscle activity in adult patients less than 65 years of age.

Comparable drugs:
OnabotulinumtoxinA (Botox), rimabotulinumtoxinB (Myobloc).

Advantages:
- May be effective in some patients in whom the benefits of other botulinum toxin products are diminished.
- Indications also include aesthetic/cosmetic use (glabellar lines) in addition to therapeutic use (compared with rimabotulinumtoxinB that has a single indication for use in patients with cervical dystonia).

Disadvantages:
- Has not been directly compared with the comparable drugs in clinical studies.
- Fewer labeled indications (compared with onabotulinumtoxinA that is also indicated for the treatment of blepharospasm and strabismus associated with dystonia, and also for the treatment of severe primary axillary hyperhidrosis).
- Formulation requires reconstitution (compared with rimabotulinumtoxinB).

Most important risks/adverse events:
Contraindicated in patients who are allergic to cow's milk protein, and in patients who have infection at the proposed injection site(s); distant spread of toxin effect (boxed warning; action of drug may spread from the area of injection and may cause swallowing and breathing difficulties that may be life-threatening); immediate medical attention may be required in cases of breathing, swallowing, or speech difficulties; clinical response may be increased in patients with concomitant neuromuscular disorders (e.g., myasthenia gravis); contains human albumin that is associated with an extremely remote risk of transmission of viral diseases and Creutzfeldt-Jakob disease; potency units are not interchangeable with other preparations of botulinum toxin products; concomitant use with aminoglycosides, muscle relaxants, or other agents that interfere with neuromuscular transmission may result in an increased response and should be closely monitored; medications with anticholinergic activity may potentiate

3

systemic anticholinergic effects; when used for glabellar lines, caution is also necessary when administering the drug in patients with surgical alterations to the facial anatomy, inflammation at the injection site, ptosis, dermatochalasis, deep dermal scarring, or thick sebaceous skin.

Most common adverse events (in patients with cervical dystonia):

Muscular weakness (16%), dysphagia (15%), dry mouth (13%), injection site discomfort (13%), fatigue (12%), headache (11%), musculoskeletal pain (7%), eye symptoms (7%), dysphonia (6%), injection site pain (5%).

Usual dosage:

Administered intramuscularly; Cervical dystonia: initially 500 units as a divided dose among the affected muscles; retreatment may be provided every 12 to 16 weeks (or longer) based on return of clinical symptoms with doses administered between 250 and 1000 units to optimize clinical benefit; titration should occur in 250 unit steps according to the patient's response; retreatment should not occur in intervals of less than 12 weeks: Glabellar lines: a total dose of 50 units, divided in 5 equal aliquots of 10 units each, is administered to affected muscles; retreatment should be administered no more frequently than every 3 months.

Products:

Cervical dystonia: single-use vials – 300 units, 500 units (to be reconstituted with preservative-free 0.9% Sodium Chloride Injection: Glabellar lines: single-use vials – 300 units; vials should be stored in a refrigerator.

Comments:

Cervical dystonia, also known as spasmodic torticollis, involves involuntary contractions of muscles of the neck, and is often associated with abnormal head position and pain. Botulinum toxin products are neuromuscular blocking toxins that have been effective in treating some patients. Following injection into the affected muscles, the toxins inhibit the release of acetylcholine from peripheral cholinergic nerve endings. This interruption of cholinergic transmission results in a localized reduction of muscle activity that gradually reverses over time. AbobotulinumtoxinA is a purified neurotoxin type A complex produced by fermentation of the bacterium Clostridium botulinum type A, Hall strain.. Vials also contain a small amount of human serum albumin and may contain trace amounts of cow's milk proteins. Its effectiveness was demonstrated in placebo-controlled studies in which the drug was administered by intramuscular injection divided among two to four affected muscles. The results in the group of patients treated with the medication were statistically significantly greater compared with those receiving placebo.

The spread of the action of the botulinum toxins that has resulted in breathing and swallowing difficulties has been reported hours to weeks after injection. The risk of such problems is thought to be greatest in children treated for spasticity but symptoms can also occur in adults, particularly in patients who have underlying conditions that predispose them to these problems.

The indications for which abobotulinumtoxinA has been approved include a therapeutic use (cervical dystonia) and an aesthetic/cosmetic use (glabellar lines; e.g., "frown lines," "crow's feet"). The Dysport products are being promoted separately for these two uses.

Acamprosate calcium (Campral – Forest)
Agent for Alcohol Dependence
2005

New Drug Comparison Rating (NDCR) = 4 (significant advantages)

Indication:
Maintenance of abstinence from alcohol in patients with alcohol dependence who are abstinent at treatment initiation.

Comparable drugs:
Disulfiram (e.g., Antabuse), naltrexone (ReVia); (naltrexone has been subsequently marketed as an extended-release injectable suspension [Vivitrol]).

Advantages:
- Unique mechanism of action (may alter gamma aminobutyric acid [GABA] and glutamate activity in a manner that restores normal neuronal balance).
- May be used safely in patients who are being treated with an opioid analgesic or who are on methadone maintenance (compared with naltrexone, which may precipitate withdrawal symptoms).
- May be used in patients with hepatic disorders (compared with naltrexone with which there may be an increased risk of hepatotoxicity).
- Does not cause unpleasant reactions if an alcoholic beverage is consumed (compared with disulfiram).

Disadvantages:
- Must be administered more frequently.

Most important risks/adverse events:
Contraindicated in patients with severe renal impairment; alcohol-dependent patients should be monitored for symptoms of depression and suicidal thinking.

Most common adverse events:
Diarrhea (17%), flatulence (4%), nausea (4%).

Usual dosage:
666 mg three times a day; dosage should be reduced in patients with moderate renal impairment.

Products:
Enteric-coated tablets – 333 mg.

Comments:

Acamprosate is the third drug approved for the treatment of alcohol dependence, joining disulfiram and naltrexone. It is structurally similar to the endogenous amino acid homotaurine which is a structural analogue of the amino acid transmitter gamma aminobutyric acid (GABA) and the amino acid neuromodulator taurine. It has been proposed that acamprosate alters GABA and glutamate activity in a way that restores normal balance between neuronal excitation and inhibition. It does not appear to exhibit other central nervous system actions, and it is not addicting. Acamprosate may be particularly useful in patients who are not candidates for naltrexone treatment (e.g., those being treated with an opioid analgesic). It should be used as part of a comprehensive management program that includes psychosocial support.

Acamprosate does not undergo metabolism and the fraction of the dose that is absorbed is primarily excreted via the kidneys in unchanged form. Its clearance is reduced in patients with moderate or severe renal impairment, and it is contraindicated in patients with severe renal impairment.

In 2007 naltrexone was marketed in an additional formulation, an extended-release injectable suspension (Vivitrol), that is administered once a month.

Alglucosidase alfa (Myozyme – Genzyme)
Agent for Pompe Disease
2006

New Drug Comparison Rating (NDCR) = 5 (important advance)

Indication:

Administered via intravenous infusion for use in patients with Pompe disease.

Comparable drugs:

None.

Advantages:

- First drug approved for Pompe disease.

Disadvantages/Limitations:

- Must be administered parenterally.
- Frequency of infusion reactions.
- Risk of hypersensitivity reactions.

Most important risks/adverse events:

Hypersensitivity reactions including anaphylactic reactions (boxed warning); risk of cardiac arrhythmia and sudden cardiac death during general anesthesia for central venous catheter placement; risk of acute cardiorespiratory failure; infusion reactions.

Most common adverse events:

Fever (92%), diarrhea (62%), rash (54%), infusion reactions (51%), vomiting (49%), cough (46%), pneumonia (46%), otitis media (44%), upper respiratory tract infection (44%), gastroenteritis (41%), decreased oxygen saturation (41%).

Usual dosage:

20 mg/kg via intravenous infusion over approximately 4 hours every 2 weeks; initial infusion rate should be no more than 1 mg/kg/hour which can be increased based on patient tolerance.

Product:

Vials – 50 mg (should be stored in a refrigerator).

Comments:

Pompe disease is a rare neuromuscular genetic disorder caused by a deficiency or dysfunction of the lysosomal hydrolase acid alpha-glucosidase that is commonly designated as GAA (for glucosidase acid alpha). The disease is also known as glycogen storage disease type II and acid maltase deficiency. The enzyme deficiency/defect results in glycogen accumulation, expansion of the lysosomes, and leakage of glycogen out of the cells, with the consequence that muscle cells are damaged and muscle function is impaired. Death is usually related to respiratory failure.

Alglucosidase alfa is human acid alpha glucosidase produced by recombinant DNA technology that provides an exogenous source of the deficient enzyme. It degrades glycogen by catalyzing the hydrolysis of glycosidic linkages of lysosomal glycogen. It has been demonstrated to improve ventilator-free survival in patients with infantile-onset Pompe disease, as compared with an untreated historical control. Experience is insufficient to assure its effectiveness and safety in patients with other forms of Pompe disease.

Aliskiren hemifumarate (Tekturna – Novartis)
Antihypertensive Agent
2007

New Drug Comparison Rating (NDCR) = 3 (no or minor advantages/disadvantages)

Indication:

Treatment of hypertension, alone or in combination with other antihypertensive agents.

Comparable drugs:

Angiotensin-converting enzyme inhibitors (ACEIs) such as lisinopril (e.g., Prinivil, Zestril); angiotensin II receptor blockers (ARBs) such as losartan (Cozaar).

Advantages:

- Unique mechanism of action (direct renin inhibitor).
- Less likely than the ACEIs to cause cough as an adverse event.

Disadvantages:

- Labeled indications are more limited (compared with the ACEIs and ARBs that have been approved for other indications [e.g., congestive heart failure] in addition to hypertension).
- Not available in a combination product with hydrochlorothiazide (has been subsequently marketed in a combination product with hydrochlorothiazide [Tekturna HCT]).
- More expensive (compared with some of the ACEIs that are available in lower cost generic formulations).

Most important risks/adverse events:

Fetal and neonatal morbidity and death if used during the second or third trimester of pregnancy (boxed warning); angioedema of the face, extremities, lips, tongue, glottis, and/or larynx; hyperkalemia, particularly if used in combination with an ACEI in patients with diabetes; action may be increased by cyclosporine (e.g., Neoral) and concurrent use is not recommended.

Most common adverse events:

Diarrhea (2%), cough (1%), hyperkalemia (1%), rash (1%).

Usual dosage:

150 mg once a day; if blood pressure is not adequately controlled, may be increased to 300 mg once a day; bioavailability may be reduced if taken with a high-fat meal and should be administered in a consistent relationship with a meal.

9

Products:

Tablets – 150 mg, 300 mg; (subsequently also marketed in combination with hydrochlorothiazide [Tekturna HCT] – 150 mg/12.5 mg, 300 mg/25 mg, and in a combination with valsartan [Valturna] – 150 mg/160 mg, 300 mg/320 mg).

Comments:

Renin is secreted by the kidney and acts on angiotensinogen to form angiotensin I. Although angiotensin I is inactive, it is converted to angiotensin II that is a potent vasoconstrictor that can increase blood pressure. The ACEIs inhibit the conversion of angiotensin I to angiotensin II, and the ARBs act at the angiotensin II receptors to reduce its action. Aliskiren is a direct renin inhibitor and is the first antihypertensive agent with this mechanism of action. Like the ACEIs and ARBs, aliskiren suppresses the negative feedback, resulting in a compensatory rise in plasma renin concentration. With the ACEIs and ARBs, this response results in increased plasma renin activity (PRA) whereas, with aliskiren, the effect of increased renin concentrations is blocked and PRA is reduced. The aliskiren-induced reductions of PRA do not correlate with blood pressure reductions and it is not known whether this difference in the effect on PRA provides any clinical advantage for aliskiren.

There are no data to demonstrate that aliskiren is either more or less effective than the ACEIs and ARBs in reducing blood pressure. In addition to hypertension, most of the ACEIs and ARBs are also indicated for the treatment of certain other cardiovascular disorders. It can be expected that additional indications will be approved for aliskiren as more studies are completed.

Alvimopan (Entereg – Adolor; GlaxoSmithKline)
Agent for Postoperative Ileus
2008

New Drug Comparison Rating (NDCR) = 4 (significant advantages)

Indication:
For short-term use in hospitalized patients to accelerate the time to upper and lower gastrointestinal recovery following large or small bowel resection surgery with primary anastomosis.

Comparable drug:
Methylnaltrexone (Relistor).

Advantages:
- Is the first drug to be demonstrated to be effective in accelerating gastrointestinal recovery following bowel resection surgery.
- Is administered orally (whereas methylnaltrexone is administered subcutaneously).

Disadvantages:
- Use is limited to short-term use in hospitalized patients.
- Effectiveness in the treatment of opioid-induced constipation has not been demonstrated.
- Available only in a restricted distribution program.

Most important risks/adverse events:
Contraindicated in patients who have taken therapeutic doses of opioids for more than 7 consecutive days immediately prior to taking alvimopan; use is limited to short-term use (15 doses) in hospitalized patients (boxed warning); a higher number of myocardial infarctions was reported in a 12-month study in patients treated with opioids for chronic pain, although a causal relationship has not been established.

Most common adverse events:
Hypokalemia (10%), dyspepsia (7%), anemia (5%), back pain (3%), urinary retention (3%); patients recently exposed to opioids may be more likely to experience adverse events.

Usual dosage:
12 mg administered 30 minutes to 5 hours prior to surgery followed by 12 mg twice a day beginning the day after surgery for a maximum of 7 days or until discharge; patients should receive no more than 15 doses, all of which should be administered while the patient is in the hospital.

Product:

Capsules – 12 mg; was approved with a Risk Evaluation and Mitigation Strategy (REMS) and is supplied only to hospitals that have registered in and meet all of the requirements for the Entereg Access Support and Education (E.A.S.E.) program.

Comments:

Following major abdominal surgery and certain other surgeries, some patients experience postoperative ileus as a result of impairment of gastrointestinal motility. This may delay recovery from the surgery and hospital discharge. Opioid analgesics are used to relieve postsurgical pain in almost all patients who have undergone major abdominal surgery; however, these agents may prolong the duration of postoperative ileus. Alvimopan is a selective antagonist of mu-opioid receptors in peripheral tissues (e.g., the gastrointestinal [GI] tract) and it antagonizes the effects of the opioid on GI motility and secretion without reversing its analgesic action that results from its action at receptors in the central nervous system. The action of alvimopan is generally similar to that of methylnaltrexone, an agent that was also approved in 2008 and marketed shortly before alvimopan. However, the indications for the two agents are different, with methylnaltrexone having been approved for the treatment of opioid-induced constipation.

Although other drugs have been used to increase gastrointestinal motility, alvimopan is the first agent to be approved to accelerate GI recovery following bowel surgery (e.g., resections necessitated by colorectal cancer). Its effectiveness was demonstrated in placebo-controlled studies in which bowel recovery times ranged from 10 to 26 hours shorter for the alvimopan-treated patients compared with the placebo-treated patients. Patients receiving alvimopan had their hospital discharge order written 13 to 21 hours sooner compared with patients receiving placebo. A higher number of myocardial infarctions was reported in a 12-month study in patients treated with opioids for chronic pain. Although a causal relationship was not established, this is the basis for a boxed warning in the labeling and restrictions regarding its distribution and dosage.

Ambrisentan (Letairis – Gilead Sciences)
Agent for Pulmonary Arterial Hypertension
2007

New Drug Comparison Rating (NDCR) = 4 (significant advantages)

Indication:
Treatment of pulmonary arterial hypertension (WHO Group 1) in patients with WHO class II or III symptoms to improve exercise capacity and delay clinical worsening.

Comparable drug:
Bosentan (Tracleer).

Advantages:
- May be satisfactorily tolerated by patients who have experienced aminotransferase elevations with the use of bosentan.
- May interact with fewer drugs.
- Administered less frequently (once a day compared with twice a day with bosentan).

Disadvantages:
- Labeled indication is more limited (indicated in patients with class II or III symptoms whereas the indication for bosentan includes patients with class III or IV symptoms).
- Has not been directly compared with bosentan.
- Available only through a restricted distribution program.

Most important risks/adverse events:
Elevations of liver aminotransferases (ALT, AST) and serious liver injury (boxed warning); may cause harm to a fetus and use is contraindicated during pregnancy (boxed warning); pregnancy must be excluded before the start of treatment and prevented thereafter by the use of two reliable methods of contraception; decreases in hemoglobin have been observed and hemoglobin should be measured at the beginning of treatment, at one month, and periodically thereafter; fluid retention; mild to moderate peripheral edema; is a substrate of CYP3A and action may be increased by the concurrent use of a CYP3A inhibitor (e.g., clarithromycin [e.g., Biaxin]), and decreased by the concurrent use of a CYP3A inducer (e.g., rifampin [e.g., Rifadin]); action may be increased by the concurrent use of cyclosporine (e.g., Neoral). Warnings and precautions regarding interactions with cyclosporine or strong CYP3A inhibitors have subsequently been deleted.

Most common adverse events:
Peripheral edema (17%), headache (15%), nasal congestion (6%), palpitations (5%), flushing (4%).

Usual dosage:

5 mg once a day, initially; if treatment is well tolerated, an increase to 10 mg once a day should be considered.

Products:

Tablets – 5 mg, 10 mg.

Comments:

Pulmonary arterial hypertension (PAH) is a rare, life-threatening condition that results from restricted blood flow to the lungs. Drugs that have been specifically approved for the treatment of PAH include epoprostenol (Flolan) and treprostinil (Remodulin) that are administered parenterally, iloprost (Ventavis) that is administered by inhalation, and bosentan and sildenafil (Revatio) that are administered orally. Tadalafil (Adcirca) has subsequently been approved for oral use for PAH.

Endothelins (ETs) are a group of peptide hormones that are released by endothelial cells, and certain of these hormones exhibit a potent vasoconstrictor action that is thought to play a critical role in the pathogenesis and worsening of PAH. Ambrisentan is an ET receptor antagonist with properties that are most similar to those of bosentan. It has a greater selectivity for ET_A receptors than bosentan, but the clinical implications of this selectivity are not known. Ambrisentan is indicated for the treatment of PAH in patients with class II or III symptoms, whereas the indication for bosentan includes patients with more serious symptoms (i.e., class III or IV symptoms). The effectiveness of ambrisentan was demonstrated in placebo-controlled studies in which it significantly improved on the 6-minute walk distance. A significant delay also was seen in the time to clinical worsening (e.g., hospitalization for PAH). The results of an uncontrolled study suggest that ambrisentan may be an appropriate option in patients with PAH who have experienced asymptomatic aminotransferase elevations with the use of bosentan.

Anidulafungin (Eraxis – Pfizer)
Antifungal Agent
2006

New Drug Comparison Rating (NDCR) = 3 (no or minor advantages/disadvantages)

Indications:
Administered via intravenous infusion for the treatment of esophageal candidiasis, and for the treatment of candidemia and other types of Candida infections (intra-abdominal abscess and peritonitis).

Comparable drugs:
Caspofungin (Cancidas), micafungin (Mycamine).

Advantages:
- Has broader labeled indications (compared with micafungin).
- Less likely to interact with cyclosporine (compared with caspofungin).

Disadvantages:
- High relapse rate in patients with esophageal candidiasis.
- Has fewer labeled indications (compared with caspofungin).

Most important risks/adverse events:
Liver function test abnormalities; histamine-mediated symptoms.

Most common adverse events:
Diarrhea (3%), hypokalemia (3%), ALT elevations (2%).

Usual dosage:
Administered via intravenous infusion at a rate that should not exceed 1.1 mg/minute (to reduce the possibility of histamine-mediated symptoms); esophageal candidiasis – 100 mg on the first day, followed by 50 mg once a day; candidemia and other Candida infections – 200 mg on the first day, followed by 100 mg once a day.

Products:
Vials – 50 mg (subsequently also marketed in vials containing 100 mg).

Comments:
Anidulafungin is the third echinocandin antifungal agent marketed in the United States, joining caspofungin and micafungin. These agents inhibit the synthesis of a glucan derivative that is an essential component of fungal cell walls but not present in

mammalian cells. They are administered via intravenous infusion and, unlike many of the azole antifungal agents, are not available in orally administered formulations.

Anidulafungin was compared with fluconazole (e.g., Diflucan) in the clinical studies. Both agents were administered intravenously in the treatment of candidemia and other Candida infections and a clinical cure or improvement was attained in 76% of the patients treated with anidulafungin and in 60% of those treated with fluconazole. In patients with esophageal candidiasis, anidulafungin was compared with the oral use of fluconazole. A cure or improvement was attained in almost all patients with both drugs; however, the relapse rate 2 weeks following the completion of therapy was much higher with anidulafungin (53%) than with fluconazole (19%).

Although the labeled indications for anidulafungin are broader than those for micafungin, they are much more limited than those for caspofungin. In addition to the indications for which anidulafungin has been approved, caspofungin is also indicated for pleural space infections caused by Candida, empiric therapy for presumed fungal infections in febrile, neutropenic patients, and invasive aspergillosis in patients who are refractory to or intolerant of other antifungal therapy.

The concurrent use of anidulafungin with cyclosporine (e.g., Neoral) is not likely to result in clinically important changes in their activity, whereas elevations of hepatic enzymes have been associated with the concurrent use of caspofungin and cyclosporine.

Artemether/lumefantrine (Coartem – Novartis)
Antiparasitic Agents
2009

New Drug Comparison Rating (NDCR) = 4 (significant advantages)

Indication:
Treatment of acute, uncomplicated malaria infections caused by Plasmodium falciparum in patients of 5 kg of bodyweight and above.

Comparable drug:
Chloroquine (e.g., Aralen).

Advantages:
- Is effective in geographical regions in which resistance to chloroquine exists.
- Effectiveness and safety have been demonstrated in young children.

Disadvantages:
- Is not indicated for malaria prophylaxis.
- May prolong the QT interval of the electrocardiogram.
- May interact with numerous other medications.

Most important risks/adverse events:
Prolongation of QT interval (use should be avoided in patients with known QT prolongation, those with hypokalemia or hypomagnesemia, those receiving other medications that prolong the QT interval [e.g., certain antiarrhythmic agents, moxifloxacin (Avelox), ziprasidone (Geodon)], and those receiving other medications with cardiac effects that are metabolized via the CYP2D6 pathway [e.g., flecainide, amitriptyline]); potential for QT prolongation may be increased by the concurrent use of CYP3A4 inhibitors (e.g., clarithromycin, grapefruit juice), halofantrine (should not be used within one month of each other), or quinine and quinidine (must be used with caution following artemether/lumefantrine); use of mefloquine (Lariam) immediately prior to treatment may reduce systemic exposure of lumefantrine; concomitant use of a substrate, inhibitor, or inducer of CYP3A4, including antiretroviral medications, may result in a loss of efficacy of the concomitant drug or additive QT prolongation; action of hormonal contraceptives may be reduced and an additional non-hormonal method of birth control should be employed.

Most common adverse events:
Adults (older than 16 years) – headache (56%), anorexia (40%), dizziness (39%), asthenia (38%), arthralgia (34%), myalgia (32%), nausea (26%), pyrexia (25%); children – pyrexia (29%), cough (23%), vomiting (18%), headache (13%), anorexia (13%).

Usual dosage:
Should be administered with food; the initial dose, followed by the second dose 8 hours later, should be administered on the first day of treatment; subsequent doses should be administered in

the morning and evening of the second and third days for a total of 6 doses; the number of tablets to be administered per dose is 4 tablets for patients weighing 35 kg or more, 3 tablets for those weighing 25 kg to less than 35 kg, 2 tablets for those weighing 15 kg to less than 25 kg, and one tablet for those weighing 5 kg to less than 15 kg; for infants, children, and other patients who are unable to swallow tablets, the tablets may be crushed and mixed with one to two teaspoonfuls of water immediately before administering the drugs.

Product:

Tablets – 20 mg artemether and 120 mg lumefantrine.

Comments:

Malaria caused by Plasmodium falciparum is resistant to chloroquine in many parts of the world. The artemisinins are derived from the leaves of the Artemisia annua plant and artemether and its active metabolite dihydroartemisinin (DHA) are among its derivatives. Although these derivatives are highly active against P. falciparum, they have a short elimination half-life that may contribute to a greater likelihood of relapse and/or faster emergence of resistance if they are used as monotherapy. Accordingly, they have been used in combination with other antimalarial agents that have a different mechanism of action. Artemether and lumefantrine have been marketed in a combination product but are not available as individual agents in the United States. Artemether is converted to the active metabolite DHA. Lumefantrine is related to halofantrine (Halfan) which is an antimalarial agent that is no longer marketed in the United States. Whereas artemether and DHA have an elimination half-life of approximately 2 hours, lumefantrine has a long terminal half-life of 3 to 6 days.

Both artemether and lumefantrine are active against the erythrocytic stages of P. falciparum, and have been approved for the treatment of acute, uncomplicated malaria infections. The combination product is not indicated for the treatment of severe malaria, for which intravenously administered antimalarial agents would be used, and it is not indicated for preventing malaria. Its effectiveness has been demonstrated in geographical regions (e.g., Thailand, Africa) in which resistance to agents such as chloroquine has been an important problem. The 28-day cure rate, defined as clearance of the erythrocytic stage within 7 days without recrudescence by day 28, was more than 95% in most studies. When artemether/lumefantrine was studied in the treatment of mixed infections caused by P. falciparum and P. vivax, all patients experienced clearing of their parasitemia within 48 hours, but parasite relapse occurred in approximately one-third of the patients. The explanation for this high rate of relapse is that, although both drugs are active against the erythrocytic stage of species of Plasmodia, they are not active against the exo-erythrocytic forms of P. vivax that exist in the liver and are the cause of subsequent relapse.

The most important concern with the use of artemether/lumefantrine is prolongation of the QT interval of the electrocardiogram and the resultant increased risk of cardiac dysrhythmias. The new product should not be used in patients with medical problems or concurrent therapy that would increase the risk of this complication.

Both artemether and lumefantrine are primarily metabolized via the CYP3A4 pathway and caution must be observed when they are used concurrently with other medications that are substrates, inhibitors, or inducers of CYP3A4. Lumefantrine may inhibit the CYP2D6 metabolic pathway and its use should be avoided in patients receiving medications that are metabolized via this pathway and have cardiac effects (e.g., flecainide).

Food, particularly a high-fat meal, significantly increases the absorption and bioavailability of both artemether and lumefantrine. Although patients with malaria often do not tolerate food well, and nausea, vomiting, and anorexia may occur as adverse events, the product should be administered with food (e.g., milk, broth, porridge, pudding, infant formula) as soon as it can be tolerated.

Asenapine (Saphris – Schering)
Antipsychotic Agent
2009

New Drug Comparison Rating (NDCR) = 2 (significant disadvantages)

Indications:

For use in adults for the acute treatment of schizophrenia and for the acute treatment of manic or mixed episodes associated with bipolar I disorder with or without psychotic features.

Comparable drug:

Olanzapine (Zyprexa).

Advantages:

- Less likely to cause weight gain.
- May interact with fewer medications.

Disadvantages:

- Has appeared to be less effective in some studies.
- Labeled indications are more limited (e.g., olanzapine has labeled indications for maintenance treatment as well as acute treatment).
- May cause QT interval prolongation (should be avoided in patients with risk factors for this response).
- Administered twice a day (whereas olanzapine is administered once a day).
- Administered sublingually.
- May cause hypoesthesia.
- Effectiveness and safety have not been established in pediatric patients (whereas olanzapine has indications for use in adolescents aged 13 to 17 years).
- Fewer formulation options (e.g., olanzapine is also available in a parenteral formulation for acute agitation and in an extended-release parenteral formulation).

Most important risks/adverse events:

Increased mortality in elderly patients with dementia-related psychosis (boxed warning; is not approved for the treatment of dementia-related psychosis); cerebrovascular adverse events; neuroleptic malignant syndrome; tardive dyskinesia; hyperglycemia and diabetes mellitus; orthostatic hypotension and syncope; QT interval prolongation (should not be used in patients at risk including those who are taking other medications that are known to cause QT prolongation [e.g., certain antiarrhythmic agents, moxifloxacin (Avelox)]); leukopenia, neutropenia, and agranulocytosis; hyperprolactinemia; disruption of body temperature regulation; dysphagia; seizures; potential for cognitive and motor impairment (patients should be cautioned about engaging in activities requiring mental alertness); suicide (risk is inherent in psychiatric illness); exposure is markedly increased in patients with severe hepatic impairment and use is not recommended in these patients; is a substrate for CYP1A2 and concurrent use with fluvoxamine (Luvox), a CYP1A2 inhibitor, should be closely monitored; may increase the action of central nervous system depressants and certain antihypertensive medications.

Most common adverse events:

Patients with schizophrenia: somnolence (13%), akathisia (6%), oral hypoesthesia (5%); Patients with bipolar disorder: somnolence (24%), dizziness (11%), extrapyramidal symptoms (excluding akathisia – 7%); increased weight (5%).

Usual dosage:

Administered sublingually; tablets should be placed under the tongue and left to dissolve completely; tablet will dissolve in saliva within seconds; patients should avoid eating and drinking for 10 minutes after administration; in patients with schizophrenia, the recommended starting and target dose is 5 mg twice a day; in patients with bipolar disorder, the recommended starting and target dose is 10 mg twice a day; the dosage may be decreased to 5 mg twice a day if there are adverse events; although a labeled indication for maintenance treatment has not yet been approved, treatment in patients who respond well to treatment may be continued beyond the acute response.

Products:

Sublingual tablets: 5 mg, 10 mg.

Comments:

Asenapine is an atypical antipsychotic agent that is classified as a dibenzo-oxepino pyrrole. Its properties are most similar to those of olanzapine, quetiapine (Seroquel), and clozapine (e.g., Clozaril). Other atypical antipsychotic agents include aripiprazole (Abilify), risperidone (e.g., Risperdal), paliperidone (Invega), and ziprasidone (Geodon). The efficacy of these agents is thought to be mediated through a combination of antagonist activity at dopamine type 2 (D2) receptors and serotonin type 2 (5-HT2) receptors. The effectiveness of asenapine in the treatment of schizophrenia was evaluated in three 6-week studies in which placebo and active controls were used. In two of the three studies asenapine demonstrated superior efficacy to placebo. However, in the third study, asenapine could not be distinguished from placebo, whereas a statistically significant difference was observed with olanzapine, the active control, although the study was not designed to directly compare the new drug with an active control. In a 52-week study, the effectiveness of asenapine was generally similar to that of olanzapine.

The effectiveness of asenapine in the treatment of bipolar disorder was evaluated in two 3-week studies in which placebo and an active control (olanzapine) were used. In one study both asenapine and olanzapine exhibited significantly greater response and remission rates compared with placebo. In the other study, the response and remission rates with asenapine were higher than those with placebo but were not considered to be significantly different, whereas the response and remission rates with olanzapine were superior to those with placebo.

In the studies in which olanzapine was used as an active control, asenapine was less likely to cause dry mouth and weight gain, but more likely to cause dizziness, nausea, akathisia, and oral hypoesthesia. In the 52-week study with asenapine, 15% of patients experienced at least a 7% increase in body weight. The effects of asenapine on the QT interval were evaluated with the use of doses up to twice the recommended dosage. The drug was associated with increases in the QTc interval ranging from 2 to 5 msec compared to placebo, but no patients experienced a QTc as high as 500 msec.

If it is administered in a conventional tablet formulation that is swallowed, the bioavailability of asenapine is very low (less than 2%). However, when administered sublingually, the bioavailability of a dose of 5 mg is 35%. Water or food may reduce asenapine exposure, and eating or drinking should be avoided for 10 minutes after administration.

Bendamustine hydrochloride (Treanda – Cephalon)
Antineoplastic Agent
2008

New Drug Comparison Rating (NDCR) = 4 (significant advantages)

Indications:
Administered intravenously for the treatment of patients with chronic lymphocytic leukemia (CLL); (has been subsequently approved for the treatment of indolent B-cell non-Hodgkin's lymphoma [NHL] that has progressed during or within six months of treatment with rituximab or a rituximab-containing regimen).

Comparable drugs (for the initial indication for CLL):
Chlorambucil (e.g., Leukeran), fludarabine (e.g., Fludara), rituximab (Rituxan).

Advantages:
- Is more effective (compared with chlorambucil in the treatment of CLL).
- Has a dual mechanism of action.

Disadvantages:
- Has not been directly compared with fludarabine and rituximab in clinical studies in patients with CLL.
- Is administered intravenously (compared with chlorambucil that is administered orally).
- More likely to interact with other medications.
- Should not be used in patients with moderate or severe hepatic impairment.

Most important risks/adverse events:
Myelosuppression (may warrant treatment delay or dose reduction); infections; infusion reactions and anaphylaxis; tumor lysis syndrome; skin reactions; other malignancies; fetal harm if used during pregnancy – Pregnancy Category D; should not be used in patients with moderate or severe hepatic impairment, or in patients with a creatinine clearance less than 40 mL/minute; is metabolized via the CYP1A2 pathway and action may be altered by the concurrent use of an inhibitor (e.g., ciprofloxacin [e.,g., Cipro]) or inducer (e.g., omeprazole [e.g., Prilosec]) of this metabolic pathway.

Most common adverse events:
Neutropenia (28%), pyrexia (24%), thrombocytopenia (23%), nausea (20%), anemia (19%), leukopenia (18%), vomiting (16%); (other adverse events reported at a frequency of 15% or higher in the studies in patients with NHL include fatigue, diarrhea, constipation, anorexia, cough, headache, weight loss, dyspnea, rash, and stomatitis).

Usual dosage:

Administered by intravenous infusion: for CLL; 100 mg/m^2 infused over 30 minutes on Days 1 and 2 of a 28-day cycle, up to 6 cycles; (for the treatment of NHL – 120 mg/m^2 infused over 60 minutes on days 1 and 2 of a 21-day cycle, up to 8 cycles).

Product:

Vials – 100 mg; contents should be reconstituted with 20 mL of Sterile Water for Injection; volume needed to provide the required dose should be immediately transferred to a 500 mL infusion bag of 0.9% Sodium Chloride Injection.

Comments:

Bendamustine is a bifunctional mechlorethamine (e.g., Mustargen) derivative with a unique structure that includes a component that acts as an alkylating agent, as well as a purine-like benzimidazole component. Although its exact mechanism of action is not known, it appears to damage the DNA in cancer cells in a manner that results in apoptosis (programmed cell death) and also acts through a nonapoptotic pathway. The effectiveness of bendamustine in the treatment of CLL was demonstrated in studies in which it was compared with chlorambucil. The overall and complete response rates with the new drug were 59% and 8%, respectively, compared with 26% and less than 1%, respectively, in patients treated with chlorambucil. The median progression-free survival was 18 months with bendamustine and 6 months with chlorambucil. For the treatment of CLL, bendamustine has not been directly compared with fludarabine and rituximab in clinical studies. (In late 2008, bendamustine was approved for an additional indication – indolent B-cell NHL that has progressed during or within 6 months of treatment with a rituximab-containing regimen. Treatment with bendamustine as a single agent resulted in an overall response rate of 74% of patients, and their disease did not progress for a median of 9.3 months.)

Benzyl alcohol (Ulesfia – Sciele)
Pediculicide
2009

New Drug Comparison Rating (NDCR) = 2 (significant disadvantages)

Indication:

Topical treatment of head lice infestation in patients 6 months of age and older.

Comparable drugs:

Permethrin (e.g., Nix), pyrethrins/piperonyl butoxide (e.g., RID).

Advantages:

- Has a unique mechanism of action (causes asphyxiation of lice).
- Is less likely to cause allergic reactions.
- Is less vulnerable to the development of resistance.

Disadvantages:

- Appears to be less effective (based on data from studies [noncomparative] of individual agents).
- Has not been directly compared with other pediculicides in clinical studies.
- Indication is more limited (compared with permethrin that is also indicated [in a higher concentration for prescription use] for the treatment of scabies, and pyrethrins/piperonyl butoxide that is also indicated for the treatment of body lice and pubic lice).
- Two treatments are needed (compared with permethrin with which one treatment is usually effective).
- Requires a prescription.

Most important risks/adverse events:

Neonatal gasping syndrome (has been reported in neonates receiving intravenous products that contain benzyl alcohol); eye exposure (eyes should be immediately flushed with water).

Most common adverse events:

Pruritus (12%), ocular irritation (6%), application site irritation (2%), application site anesthesia and hypoesthesia (2%).

Usual dosage:

Product labeling should be consulted for the guidelines for the amount of lotion to be used per treatment that are based on the length of the hair; patients with medium-length hair (4 to 16 inches) may need up to 3 bottles of lotion and those with long hair may need up to 6 bottles; lotion should be applied to dry hair in a quantity sufficient to completely saturate the scalp and hair; after 10 minutes, the lotion should be completely rinsed off with water; after the lotion is washed off the hair, a fine-tooth comb may be used to remove dead lice and nits from the hair and scalp; a second treatment should be applied one week after the first treatment.

Product:

Lotion – 5%.

Comments:

For many years benzyl alcohol has been included as a component of numerous nonprescription combination products that are applied topically, and has also been used as an excipient in some solutions that are administered intravenously. However, most recently it has been evaluated for therapeutic use as a pediculicide and its approval for this purpose is the basis for its being designated as a "new" drug. Benzyl alcohol is thought to inhibit lice from closing their respiratory spiracles, thereby allowing the lotion vehicle to obstruct the spiracles and causing the lice to asphyxiate. It is likely that this mechanism of action makes it less vulnerable to the development of resistance. Benzyl alcohol does not have ovicidal activity.

The effectiveness of benzyl alcohol was demonstrated in two vehicle-controlled studies in which the lotion was applied twice (one week apart). In both studies approximately 75% of patients were free of live lice 14 days after the second treatment. Benzyl alcohol has not been directly compared with other pediculicides in clinical studies. However, experience with the comparable drugs has usually been associated with successful treatment in more than 90% of patients although increasing resistance has been recently reported.

Benzyl alcohol lotion should be used as part of an overall lice management program. All recently worn clothing and hats, as well as bedding and towels, should be washed in hot water or dry-cleaned. Personal care items such as combs, brushes, and hair clips should be washed in hot water.

Bepotastine besilate (Bepreve – Ista)
Agent for Allergic Conjunctivitis
2009

New Drug Comparison Rating (NDCR) = 2 (significant disadvantages)

Indication:

Treatment of itching associated with signs and symptoms of allergic conjunctivitis.

Comparable drugs:

Ophthalmic agents with both antihistamine and mast cell-stabilizing actions – azelastine (Optivar), epinastine (Elestat), ketotifen (Alaway, Zaditor), olopatadine (Pataday, Patanol).

Advantages:

- None.

Disadvantages:

- Administered twice a day (compared with the 0.2% concentration of olopatadine [Pataday] that is administered once a day).
- Requires a prescription (compared with ketotifen that is available without a prescription).

Most important risks/adverse events:

Should not be used to treat contact lens-related irritation; contact lenses should be removed prior to instillation.

Most common adverse events:

Mild taste (25%), other adverse events occurring in 2% to 5% of patients – eye irritation, headache, nasopharyngitis.

Usual dosage:

One drop in the affected eye(s) twice a day.

Product:

Ophthalmic solution – 1.5%.

Comments:

The effectiveness of bepotastine was demonstrated in two studies in which it was more effective than its vehicle for relieving ocular itching induced by an ocular allergen challenge. It has not been directly compared in clinical studies with other antihistamines and/or mast cell stabilizers.

Like many other ophthalmic solution formulations, bepotastine ophthalmic solution contains benzalkonium chloride as a preservative. This agent may be absorbed by soft contact lenses, and contact lenses should be removed prior to instillation of bepotastine ophthalmic solution. They may be reinserted after 10 minutes following its administration.

Besifloxacin hydrochloride (Besivance – Bausch & Lomb)
Antibacterial Agent
2009

New Drug Comparison Rating (NDCR) = 3 (no or minor advantages/disadvantages)

Indication:
For ophthalmic administration for the treatment of bacterial conjunctivitis caused by susceptible isolates of the following bacteria: CDC Corynebacterium group G, Corynebacterium pseudodiphtheriticum*, Corynebacterium striatum*, Haemophilus influenzae, Moraxella lacunata*, Staphylococcus aureus, Staphylococcus epidermidis, Staphylococcus hominis*, Staphylococcus lugdunensis*, Streptococcus mitis group, Streptococcus oralis, Streptococcus pneumoniae, Streptococcus salivarius* (efficacy against bacteria designated with an asterisk was demonstrated in fewer than 10 infections).

Comparable drugs:
Ophthalmic fluoroquinolones: Ciprofloxacin (e.g., Ciloxan), ofloxacin (e.g., Ocuflox), levofloxacin (e.g., Quixin), gatifloxacin (Zymar), and moxifloxacin (Vigamox).

Advantages:
- Effectiveness in the treatment of bacterial conjunctivitis has been demonstrated against a larger number of bacteria.
- Is administered less frequently (three times a day, compared with ciprofloxacin, gatifloxacin, levofloxacin, and ofloxacin).

Disadvantages:
- Has not been directly compared with other ophthalmic fluoroquinolones in clinical studies.
- Labeled indications are more limited (compared with ciprofloxacin, levofloxacin, and ofloxacin that are also indicated for the treatment of corneal ulcers).
- Is available in fewer formulation options (compared with ciprofloxacin that is also available in an ophthalmic ointment).

Most important risks/adverse events:
Prolonged use may result in superinfection; patients should not wear contact lenses if they have signs or symptoms of bacterial conjunctivitis, or during the course of treatment with besifloxacin.

Most common adverse events:
Conjunctival redness (2%).

Usual dosage:

One drop in the affected eye(s) 3 times a day, 4 to 12 hours apart, for 7 days.

Product:

Ophthalmic suspension – 0.6%; bottle should be inverted and shaken once prior to each dose.

Comments:

Bacterial conjunctivitis, often referred to as "pink eye," is one of the most common eye infections that usually continues for 7 to 14 days. Besifloxacin is the sixth fluoroquinolone to be marketed for ophthalmic use in the treatment of bacterial conjunctivitis but, unlike its predecessors, it is not also marketed in other formulations for the treatment of systemic infections. The new drug has been demonstrated to be effective against a larger number of specific bacteria than the other fluoroquinolones, but certain of the older drugs have been demonstrated to be effective in the treatment of bacterial conjunctivitis caused by bacteria for which the efficacy of besifloxacin has not been established (e.g., ofloxacin for infection caused by Pseudomonas aeruginosa, moxifloxacin for infection caused by Chlamydia trachomatis).

The effectiveness of besifloxacin was demonstrated in clinical studies in which the drug was compared with its vehicle. Patients treated with the drug experienced a faster rate of resolution of the infection. Clinical resolution of the infection was achieved in 45% of those receiving the drug compared with 33% of those treated with the vehicle. Microbiological outcomes demonstrated eradication rates for the causative pathogens of 91% and 60%, respectively, in the drug and vehicle treated groups, although microbiologic eradication does not always correlate with clinical outcomes. Besifloxacin has not been directly compared with other fluoroquinolones in clinical studies.

The safety of besifloxacin has been demonstrated in children as young as one year of age.

Bismuth subcitrate potassium
(Pylera [with metronidazole and tetracycline] – Axcan)
Antiulcer Agent
2007

New Drug Comparison Rating (NDCR) = 3 (no or minor advantages/disadvantages)

Indication:
In combination with omeprazole for the treatment of patients with Helicobacter pylori infection and duodenal ulcer disease (active or history of within the past five years) to eradicate H. pylori.

Comparable drugs:
Helidac regimen (bismuth subsalicylate [Pepto-Bismol], metronidazole, and tetracycline, in conjunction with an H2-receptor antagonist); regimen including omeprazole, amoxicillin, and clarithromycin; regimen including lansoprazole, amoxicillin, and clarithromycin (PrevPac).

Advantages:
- May be used in patients who are allergic to penicillins (compared with amoxicillin-containing regimens).
- Shorter duration of treatment (10 days compared with 14 days with the Helidac regimen).
- Bismuth salt is swallowed in capsule (compared with tablet in the Helidac regimen that is chewed).

Disadvantages:
- Less convenient dosage regimen (administered four times a day compared with twice a day with the amoxicillin/clarithromycin-containing regimens).

Most important risks/adverse events:
Neurotoxicity (associated with excessive doses); may interfere with diagnostic imaging of the gastrointestinal tract (because bismuth absorbs x-rays); contraindications, warnings, and precautions with metronidazole and tetracycline must also be observed.

Most common adverse events:
Stool abnormality (16%; black stool attributable to bismuth), diarrhea (9%), abdominal pain (9%), dyspepsia (9%), darkening of the tongue.

Usual dosage:

Three capsules (representing 420 mg of bismuth subcitrate potassium, 375 mg of metronidazole, and 375 mg of tetracycline) four times a day after meals and at bedtime for 10 days; used in conjunction with omeprazole for which the recommended dosage is 20 mg twice a day after the morning and evening meals for 10 days.

Product:

Capsules containing 125 mg of tetracycline in an inner capsule and a blend of 140 mg of bismuth subcitrate potassium and 125 mg of metronidazole in the outer area of the larger capsule.

Comments:

Bismuth subcitrate potassium, also known as biskalcitrate, is a soluble, complex bismuth salt of citric acid. It is not available as a single agent but is included in a combination formulation (Pylera) that also includes metronidazole and tetracycline. This formulation is used in conjunction with omeprazole in a "quadruple" regimen that is most similar in content to the Helidac regimen. In the clinical studies, the Pylera regimen was compared with an omeprazole/amoxicillin/clarithromycin regimen and was at least as effective as the latter regimen in eradicating Helicobacter pylori in patients with duodenal ulcer disease. The Pylera regimen is most useful in patients who are allergic to penicillins and in patients in whom clarithromycin-containing regimens have not been effective.

Although bismuth is presumed to reduce the absorption of tetracycline, the clinical importance of reduced tetracycline systemic exposure is not known because the relative contribution of systemic versus local antimicrobial activity against H. pylori has not been established. Bismuth subcitrate potassium and tetracyciine are physically separated in the capsule formulation in which they are supplied by placing tetracycline in an inner capsule that is contained within a larger capsule that contains a blend of the bismuth salt and metronidazole in the outer area.

C1 Inhibitor (Human) (Cinryze – ViroPharma)
Agent for Hereditary Angioedema
2008

New Drug Comparison Rating (NDCR) = 5 (important advance)

Indication:
Administered intravenously for routine prophylaxis against angioedema attacks in adolescent and adult patients with hereditary angioedema.

Comparable drug:
Danazol.

Advantages:
- Has a unique mechanism of action.
- Less likely to cause serious adverse events.

Disadvantages:
- Must be administered intravenously (danazol is administered orally).

Most important risks/adverse events:
Hypersensitivity reactions (epinephrine should be immediately available); thrombotic events; infections (product is made from human plasma and may contain infectious agents such as viruses and, theoretically, the Creutzfeldt-Jakob disease agent).

Most common adverse events (occurring at an incidence of 5% or higher):
Upper respiratory tract infection, sinusitis, rash, headache.

Usual dosage:
Administered via intravenous infusion; 1,000 units every 3 or 4 days at an infusion rate of 1 mL/minute.

Product:
Vials – 500 units (should be protected from light); two vials of reconstituted drug are combined for a single dose; each vial is reconstituted with 5 mL of Sterile Water for Injection; each vial contains 5 mL of solution with a drug concentration of 100 units/mL.

Comments:
Hereditary angioedema (HAE) is a severely debilitating, life-threatening genetic disorder that is caused by a deficiency of C1-esterase inhibitor (C1 inhibitor), a human plasma protein. C1 inhibitor regulates the contact, complement, and fibrinolytic systems

which, if insufficiently restricted, may initiate or exacerbate attacks of inflammation. Patients with C1 inhibitor deficiency may experience unpredictable, recurrent, and potentially life-threatening attacks of inflammation of the larynx, face, abdomen, extremities, and urogenital tract. Asphyxiation may occur as a consequence of swelling of the larynx. Danazol and anabolic steroids have been used to prevent HAE attacks but these agents have been of limited effectiveness and have been associated with the occurrence of serious adverse events.

C1 inhibitor (Human) is a sterile lyophilized preparation derived from human plasma that is manufactured using a sequence of steps (e.g., pasteurization [heat treatment], nanofiltration) to reduce the risk of viral transmission. Administration of the drug increases plasma levels of C1 inhibitor activity and its effectiveness was evaluated in a placebo-controlled study. Patients treated with C1 inhibitor had a 66% reduction in days of swelling, as well as decreases in the average severity of attacks and the average duration of attacks. The approval of C1 inhibitor is for the prevention of HAE attacks. Studies of its use for the treatment of HAE attacks are being conducted but this is not a labeled indication at the present time. Another C1 inhibitor product (Berinert) was marketed in 2009 for the treatment of acute abdominal or facial attacks of HAE in adult and adolescent patients.

Canakinumab (Ilaris – Novartis)
Agent for Cryopyrin-Associated Periodic Syndromes
2009

New Drug Comparison Rating (NDCR) = 4 (significant advantages)

Indications:
Administered subcutaneously for the treatment of Cryopyrin-Associated Periodic Syndromes (CAPS), in adults and children 4 years of age and older including Familial Cold Autoinflammatory Syndrome (FCAS) and Muckle-Wells Syndrome (MWS).

Comparable drug:
Rilonacept (Arcalyst).

Advantages:
- Administered less frequently (every 8 weeks compared with every week with rilonacept).
- Effectiveness and safety have been demonstrated in children as young as 4 years of age (compared with 12 years of age with rilonacept).

Disadvantages:
- Should be administered by a healthcare provider (compared with self-administration with rilonacept).

Most important risks/adverse events:
Increased risk of infection (treatment should not be initiated in patients with an active infection; in patients being treated with canakinumab, treatment should be discontinued if a serious infection develops); concurrent use with a tumor necrosis factor (TNF) inhibitor (e.g., etanercept [Enbrel]) or the interleukin-1 (IL-1) blocker anakinra (Kineret) should be avoided because of the increased risk of infection; live vaccines should not be used during treatment, and patients should receive all recommended vaccinations before being treated with the drug.

Most common adverse events:
Nasopharyngitis (34%), diarrhea (20%), influenza (17%), rhinitis (17%), headache (14%), nausea (14%).

Usual dosage:
Administered subcutaneously every 8 weeks; recommended dosage is 150 mg for patients with body weight greater than 40 kg; for patients with body weight between 15 and 40 kg, the recommended dose is 2 mg/kg; for children 15 to 40 kg with an inadequate response, the dose can be increased to 3 mg/kg.

Product:

Vials – 180 mg; should be stored in a refrigerator; lyophilized powder is reconstituted with 1 mL of preservative-free Sterile Water for Injection.

Comments:

CAPS are a group of rare, inherited chronic inflammatory diseases that are characterized, in part, by symptoms such as recurrent rash, fever/chills, joint pain, fatigue, and eye pain/redness. CAPS include three related disorders, FCAS, MWS, and neonatal-onset multisystem inflammatory disease (NOMID). The symptoms of FCAS are triggered by exposure to cooling temperatures, and MWS symptoms are triggered by random, unknown factors and possibly exercise, stress, and cold. CAPS are generally caused by mutations in the NLRP-3 (nucleotide-binding domain, leucine-rich family [NLR], pyrin domain containing 3) gene, which encodes cryopyrin, a protein that regulates inflammation in the body. The mutation in the NLRP-3 gene causes increased activity of cryopyrin, which causes an overproduction of interleukin (IL)-1 beta, resulting in an inflammatory response and the symptoms of CAPS.

Rilonacept is an IL-1 blocker that was marketed in 2008 as the first medication to be approved for the treatment of CAPS. Canakinumab is a human monoclonal anti-human IL-1 beta antibody that neutralizes the activity of IL-1 beta by blocking its interaction with IL-1 receptors. The effectiveness of canakinumab was demonstrated in a study in which a complete response was observed in 71% of patients one week following initiation of treatment and in 97% of patients by week 8. Patients achieving a complete clinical response were randomized into a placebo-controlled withdrawal period as the second part of this study. A total of 81% of the patients randomized to placebo experienced a flare of the disease compared to none (0%) of the patients randomized to canakinumab. The drug provides a long-lasting benefit and is administered every 8 weeks, compared with weekly administration with rilonacept.

Certolizumab pegol (Cimzia – UCB)
Agent for Crohn's Disease
2008

New Drug Comparison Rating (NDCR) = 3 (no or minor advantages/disadvantages)

Indication:
Administered subcutaneously for reducing the signs and symptoms of Crohn's disease and maintaining clinical response in adult patients with moderately to severely active disease who have had an inadequate response to conventional therapy. Subsequently approved in 2009 for the treatment of adults with moderately to severely active rheumatoid arthritis.

Comparable drugs:
Adalimumab (Humira); infliximab (Remicade).

Advantages:
- Less frequent administration (compared with adalimumab that is administered every two weeks).
- Is administered subcutaneously (compared with infliximab that is administered intravenously).
- May be less likely to cause injection site reactions (compared with adalimumab).

Disadvantages:
- Labeled indication is more limited (indication does not include inducing and maintaining clinical remission).
- Has not been directly compared with other agents in clinical studies.
- Fewer labeled indications (adalimumab and infliximab also have other labeled indications [e.g., rheumatoid arthritis, psoriatic arthritis, plaque psoriasis, ankylosing spondylitis])(has been subsequently approved for rheumatoid arthritis).
- More frequent administration (compared with infliximab that is administered every eight weeks).
- Each dose should be administered as two injections by a health professional (compared with adalimumab that may be self-administered as a single injection).
- Is not indicated for use in pediatric patients (compared with infliximab).

Most important risks/adverse events:
Serious infections (boxed warning; e.g., tuberculosis, invasive fungal infections, and other opportunistic infections [patients should be evaluated for tuberculosis risk factors and be tested for latent tuberculosis infection; treatment should not be initiated in patients with active infections including chronic or localized infections; treatment should be discontinued if a patient develops a serious infection]); concurrent use with anakinra

(Kineret) is not recommended; malignancies (boxed warning was added in 2009 regarding the risk of lymphoma and other malignancies in children and adolescents); exacerbation or new onset of demyelinating disease; exacerbation or new onset of congestive heart failure; lupus-like syndrome; hepatitis B virus reactivation; hypersensitivity reactions; hematological reactions; live or attenuated vaccines should not be use concurrently.

Most common adverse events:

Upper respiratory tract infection (20%), urinary tract infection (7%), arthralgia (6%).

Usual dosage:

400 mg (administered as two subcutaneous injections of 200 mg) initially, and at weeks 2 and 4; in patients who obtain a clinical response, the recommended maintenance dosage is 400 mg every 4 weeks.

Product:

Vials – 200 mg (should be stored in a refrigerator); doses should be prepared and administered by a health professional.

Comments:

Certolizumab pegol is a recombinant, humanized antibody Fab fragment that is conjugated to a polyethylene glycol. It binds to tumor necrosis factor alpha (TNF alpha) and is the third of the TNF blockers to be approved for the treatment of patients with Crohn's disease, joining infliximab and adalimumab. However, whereas the labeled indication for the latter two agents includes maintaining clinical remission, the indication for certolizumab includes maintaining a clinical response that reflects a less pronounced effect as determined using a Crohn's Disease Activity Index. The effectiveness of the new drug was demonstrated in placebo-controlled studies; it has not been compared directly with other agents in clinical studies. The risks and adverse events associated with certolizumab are generally similar to those of adalimumab, infliximab, and the other TNF blockers, and include the risk of serious infections. Like adalimumab, certolizumab is administered subcutaneously.

Ciclesonide (Omnaris; Alvesco – Nycomed; Sepracor)
Corticosteroid
2008

New Drug Comparison Rating (NDCR) = 3 (no or minor advantages/disadvantages)

Indication:

Administered intranasally (Omnaris) for the treatment of nasal symptoms associated with seasonal allergic rhinitis in adults and children 6 years of age and older, and for the treatment of nasal symptoms associated with perennial allergic rhinitis in adults and adolescents 12 years of age and older; (subsequently approved for oral inhalation [Alvesco] for the maintenance treatment of asthma as prophylactic therapy in adult and adolescents 12 years of age and older).

Comparable drugs (for the initial indication of allergic rhinitis):

Corticosteroids in nasal spray formulations: Beclomethasone dipropionate (Beconase AQ), budesonide (Rhinocort Aqua), flunisolide (e.g., Nasarel), fluticasone furoate (Veramyst), fluticasone propionate (e.g., Flonase), mometasone furoate (Nasonex), triamcinolone acetonide (Nasacort AQ).

Advantages:

- Administered once a day (compared with beclomethasone dipropionate that is administered twice a day and flunisolide that is administered two or three times a day).

Disadvantages:

- Has not been directly compared with other intranasal corticosteroids in clinical studies.
- Labeled indications are more limited (compared with beclomethasone dipropionate. that is also indicated for nonallergic rhinitis and for the prevention of recurrence of nasal polyps following surgical removal, fluticasone propionate that is also indicated for nonallergic rhinitis, and mometasone furoate that is also indicated for prophylaxis of nasal symptoms of seasonal allergic rhinitis and the treatment of nasal polyps).
- Use in pediatric patients is more limited (compared with fluticasone furoate and mometasone furoate [and subsequently triamcinolone acetonide] that are indicated for the treatment of seasonal and perennial rhinitis in children as young as 2 years of age and fluticasone propionate that is indicated in children as young as 4 years of age).
- More expensive than intranasal corticosteroids that are available in generic formulations (flunisolide, fluticasone propionate).

Most important risks/adverse events:

Risk of acute adrenal insufficiency if a systemic corticosteroid is discontinued and replaced with a topical (e.g., nasal) corticosteroid such as ciclesonide; suppression of the immune system increases susceptibility to infection; immediate hypersensitivity reactions have been rarely reported; may delay wound healing in patients who have had recent nasal surgery or nasal septal ulcers (should not be used until healing has occurred); patients who are treated for several months or longer should be examined periodically for evidence of Candida infection; may cause a reduction in growth velocity when administered to pediatric patients; (Formulation for oral inhalation is also contraindicated in patients with status asthmaticus or other acute episodes of asthma; may cause Candida albicans infections of the mouth and pharynx [patients should be advised to rinse mouth following inhalation]; possible development of glaucoma, increased intraocular pressure, and posterior subcapsular cataracts).

Most common adverse events (in patients aged 12 years and older):

Nasal spray - headache (6%), epistaxis (5%), nasopharyngitis (4%), ear pain (2%); Oral inhalation (160 mcg twice a day) – headache (11%), nasopharyngitis (9%), upper respiratory infection (9%), sinusitis (6%), nasal congestion (6%) .

Usual dosage:

Nasal spray - 200 mcg per day administered as 2 sprays (50 mcg/spray) in each nostril once a day; Oral inhalation – 160 (80 – 320) mcg twice a day.

Product:

Nasal spray – 50 mcg/spray; is a metered dose, pump spray containing 120 metered doses; following removal from the foil pouch in which it is supplied, the bottle should be discarded either after 120 sprays following initial priming or after 4 months; bottle should be shaken gently prior to administration; before the first use, the pump should be primed by pressing on the applicator eight times; Oral inhalation aerosol – 80 mcg/actuation, 160 mcg/actuation.

Comments:

Ciclesonide is a prodrug that is enzymatically hydrolyzed by esterases in the nasal mucosa to a pharmacologically active metabolite, des-ciclesonide. Its effectiveness in the treatment of seasonal and perennial allergic rhinitis has been established in placebo-controlled studies, but it has not been directly compared with other intranasal corticosteroids in clinical studies. The onset of effect was seen within 24 to 48 hours with further symptomatic improvement observed over 1 to 2 weeks in seasonal allergic rhinitis and five weeks in perennial allergic rhinitis.

Ciclesonide was initially approved in October 2006 but was not marketed until 2008. Its initial approval for use in patients 12 years of age and older was expanded in 2007 to include children 6 to 11 years with seasonal allergic rhinitis. In early 2008 a formulation for oral inhalation was approved for the maintenance treatment of asthma and this formulation was marketed in late 2008.

Clevidipine butyrate (Cleviprex — The Medicines Company)
Antihypertensive Agent
2008

New Drug Comparison Rating (NDCR) = 3 (no or minor advantages/disadvantages)

Indication:
For intravenous use for the reduction of blood pressure when oral therapy is not feasible or not desirable.

Comparable drug:
Nicardipine (Cardene IV).

Advantages:
- Short duration of action permits more "minute-to-minute" control of blood pressure.
- Less likely to interact with other drugs.

Disadvantages:
- Not available in an orally-administered formulation.
- Short duration of action requires closer monitoring.
- Use is contraindicated in patients who are allergic to egg or soy products.
- Use is contraindicated in patients with defective lipid metabolism.
- Dosage may be limited by lipid load restrictions.

Most important risks/adverse events:
Emulsion formulation contains soybean oil, purified egg yolk phospholipids, and glycerin, and use is contraindicated in patients with a history of allergy to soybeans, soy products, eggs, or egg products; contraindicated in patients with defective lipid metabolism and in patients with severe aortic stenosis; other risks include systemic hypotension, reflex tachycardia, negative inotropic effects, exacerbation of heart failure (patients with heart failure should be closely monitored), acute renal failure, and atrial fibrillation.

Most common adverse events:
Atrial fibrillation (21% [12% with placebo]), nausea (21% [12% with placebo]), acute renal failure (9%).

Usual dosage:
Administered by intravenous infusion and is titrated to attain the desired blood pressure reduction; initial dosage is 1-2 mg/hour which then may be doubled at short (90 second) intervals; as the blood pressure approaches goal, the increase in doses should be less than

doubling and the time between dose adjustments should be lengthened to every 5-10 minutes; for most patients the desired therapeutic response occurs at doses of 4-6 mg/hour; because of lipid load restrictions, no more than 1000 mL of clevidipine infusion should be administered in a 24-hour period.

Product:

Premixed single-use vials – 0.5 mg/mL in a milky-white, oil-in-water emulsion vehicle (should be stored in a refrigerator); vials should be kept in their cartons to protect against photodegradation.

Comments:

Clevidipine is a dihydropyridine calcium channel blocker with properties and uses that can best be compared with those of nicardipine (Cardene IV). Both of these agents are administered intravenously for the reduction of blood pressure when oral therapy is not feasible or not desirable; nicardipine is also available in a capsule formulation (Cardene SR) for oral use. Clevidipine is most useful for the urgent treatment of hypertension (e.g., perioperative hypertension, severe hypertension). Like nicardipine, it has a rapid onset of action (2-4 minutes); however, the new drug has a much shorter duration of action (usually less than 15 minutes) than nicardipine (at least 3 hours). The short duration of action requires closer monitoring but permits more rapid adjustments of the blood pressure-lowering response than is possible with longer-acting agents. The effectiveness of clevidipine in the treatment of perioperative hypertension was demonstrated in two placebo-controlled studies. The target decrease in blood pressure was attained in more than 90% of patients, with marked lowering of blood pressure occurring in most patients within 5 minutes. In three studies patients received clevidipine or nicardipine, nitroglycerin, or sodium nitroprusside. Blood pressure control was similar with all four agents.

Clevidipine is rapidly metabolized to inactive metabolites by esterases in the blood and extravascular tissues. Its elimination is not significantly affected by hepatic or renal dysfunction.

Clofarabine (Clolar – Genzyme)
Antineoplastic Agent
2005

New Drug Comparison Rating (NDCR) = 4 (significant advantages)

Indications:

Administered via intravenous infusion for the treatment of pediatric patients 1 to 21 years of age with relapsed or refractory acute lymphoblastic leukemia (ALL) after at least two prior regimens.

Comparable drugs (for use in treating ALL):

e.g., cytarabine (e.g., Cytosar-U), doxorubicin (e.g., Adriamycin), asparaginase (Elspar), pegaspargase (Oncaspar), mercaptopurine (e.g., Purinethol), methotrexate (e.g., Trexall), teniposide (Vumon), vincristine (e.g., Vincasar).

Advantages:

• May provide remissions in patients who are refractory to or who relapsed with other treatment.

Disadvantages:

• Clinical benefit (e.g., prolonged survival) has not yet been documented (approved under the provisions of the accelerated approval process based on the induction of complete responses).
• Not indicated for first-line treatment for ALL.

Most important risks/adverse events:

Myelosuppression (e.g., neutropenia, anemia, thrombocytopenia); tumor lysis syndrome; systemic inflammatory response syndrome (SIRS); capillary leak syndrome; dehydration; hypotension; elevations of hepatic function tests; may cause harm to a fetus if administered during pregnancy.

Most common adverse events:

Vomiting (83%), nausea (75%), neutropenia (57%), diarrhea (53%), pruritus (47%), headache (46%), dermatitis (41%), pyrexia (41%), elevations of ALT and AST (40%), rigors (38%), fatigue (36%), abdominal pain (36%), hypotension (29%).

Usual dosage:

Administered as an intravenous infusion over a period of 2 hours; 52 mg/m^2 once a day for 5 consecutive days; treatment cycles are repeated following recovery or return to baseline organ function, approximately every 2 to 6 weeks.

Product:

Vials – 20 mg (in 20 mL of 0.9% Sodium Chloride Injection); solution should be filtered through a sterile 0.2 micrometer syringe filter and then further diluted with 0.9% Sodium Chloride Injection or 5% Dextrose Injection.

Comments:

Acute lymphoblastic leukemia (ALL) is the most common form of pediatric leukemia, and children who do not respond to initial treatment, or who experience a relapse, have a poor prognosis. Clofarabine is a purine nucleoside antimetabolite that is most similar structurally to cladribine (Leustatin) and fludarabine (Fludara) although these agents are not indicated for the treatment of pediatric ALL. Clofarabine is metabolized intracellularly to its active triphosphate metabolite that inhibits DNA synthesis. In the clinical studies there was a 30% response rate with clofarabine, with 20% of patients experiencing a complete response and 10% a partial response. Most of these patients had received 2 to 4 prior regimens, and clofarabine represents a valuable addition to the group of agents that may be of benefit in the treatment of pediatric ALL.

Severe bone marrow suppression is the most important concern associated with the use of clofarabine, and patients are at increased risk for severe opportunistic infections as well. Complete blood and platelet counts should be determined at regular intervals during treatment. Patients should also be monitored for signs and symptoms of tumor lysis syndrome, as well as cytokine release (e.g., tachypnea, tachycardia, hypotension) that could develop into SIRS/capillary leak syndrome, and organ dysfunction. Continuous administration of intravenous fluids is recommended throughout the 5 days of clofarabine use.

Conivaptan hydrochloride (Vaprisol – Astellas)
Agent for Hyponatremia
2006

New Drug Comparison Rating (NDCR) = 5 (important advance)

Indications:
Administered via intravenous infusion for the treatment of euvolemic hyponatremia in hospitalized patients; (subsequently approved for the treatment of hypervolemic hyponatremia in hospitalized patients).

Comparable drugs:
None (Tolvaptan [Samsca] was subsequently marketed in 2009).

Advantages:
- First drug approved for the treatment of euvolemic hyponatremia.
- Unique mechanism of action (arginine vasopressin antagonist).

Disadvantages/Limitations:
- Must be administered as a continuous intravenous infusion.
- Risk of neurologic adverse events.

Most important risks/adverse events:
Contraindicated in patients with hypovolemic hyponatremia; is a substrate of CYP3A4 and concurrent use of a potent CYP3A4 inhibitor (e.g., clarithromycin [e.g., Biaxin]) is contraindicated; overly rapid correction of serum sodium may result in serious neurologic sequelae (neurologic status should be monitored); injection site reactions; inhibits CYP3A4 and may increase the action of other medications that are metabolized via this metabolic pathway (e.g., simvastatin [e.g., Zocor]).

Most common adverse events:
Infusion site reactions (20%), infusion site phlebitis (16%), infusion site pain (8%), headache (12%), thirst (10%), hypokalemia (10%).

Usual dosage:
Administered by intravenous infusion using large veins; treatment is initiated with a loading dose of 20 mg administered over 30 minutes; loading dose is followed by a dose of 20 mg administered in a continuous intravenous infusion over 24 hours; following the first day of treatment, should be administered for an additional 1 to 3 days in a continuous infusion of 20 mg per day; if the serum sodium concentration is not increasing at the desired rate, the dosage may be titrated upward to a dose of 40 mg per

day in a continuous intravenous infusion; the total duration of infusion (after the loading dose) should not exceed 4 days; infusion site should be changed every 24 hours to reduce the risk of vascular irritation.

Product:

Ampules – 20 mg (in 4 mL of solution); drug should be diluted only with 5% Dextrose Injection and should not be mixed or administered with 0.9% Sodium Chloride Injection or Lactated Ringer's Injection.

Comments:

Dilutional hyponatremia is the most common form of hyponatremia and occurs when total body water increases, thereby diluting serum sodium concentrations. The hormone arginine vasopressin (AVP), previously referred to as the antidiuretic hormone, regulates water loss from the body by altering water permeability of the renal collecting ducts, primarily by acting at V2 receptors. Dilutional hyponatremia can be further classified as euvolemic or hypervolemic, depending on the volume status of the patient. Euvolemic hyponatremia is commonly associated with the syndrome of inappropriate secretion of antidiuretic hormone (SIADH) that is often present in endocrine disorders, and hypervolemic hyponatremia is often associated with underlying conditions such as congestive heart failure.

Conivaptan was initially approved for the treatment of euvolemic hyponatremia (e.g., SIADH, or in the setting of hypothyroidism, adrenal insufficiency, pulmonary disorders) in hospitalized patients, and is the first drug to be approved for this indication. It was subsequently approved for the treatment of hypervolemic hyponatremia in hospitalized patients. It acts as a dual AVP antagonist and has affinity for both V2 and V1A receptors. Its primary action is V2 antagonism of AVP in the renal collecting ducts. Its effectiveness in increasing serum sodium concentrations was demonstrated in placebo-controlled studies.

Darifenacin hydrobromide (Enablex – Novartis)
Agent for Overactive Bladder
2005

New Drug Comparison Rating (NDCR) = 3 (no or minor advantages/disadvantages)

Indication:
Treatment of overactive bladder with symptoms of urge urinary incontinence, urgency, and urinary frequency.

Comparable drugs:
Oxybutynin (e.g., Ditropan XL), solifenacin (Vesicare), tolterodine (Detrol LA), trospium (Sanctura).

Advantages:
- Administered once a day (compared with trospium that is administered twice a day).
- Does not appear to prolong the QT interval (compared with solifenacin, which has been reported to do so).

Disadvantages:
- May interact with more medications (as a result of being metabolized via two major metabolic pathways—CYP3A4 and CYP2D6).

Most important risks/adverse events:
Contraindicated in patients with urinary retention, gastric retention, or uncontrolled narrow-angle glaucoma, and in patients who are at risk of these conditions; is extensively metabolized (primarily via the CYP3A4 and CYP2D6 pathways) and its action may be significantly increased by the concurrent use of a potent CYP3A4 inhibitor (e.g., clarithromycin [e.g., Biaxin]); is not recommended for use in patients with severe hepatic impairment.

Most common adverse events:
Dry mouth (20%), constipation (15%), dyspepsia (3%)—incidences reported are with a dosage of 7.5 mg once a day and are higher with a dosage of 15 mg once a day.

Usual dosage:
7.5 mg once a day, initially; if satisfactorily tolerated, may be increased to 15 mg once a day; dosage should not exceed 7.5 mg once a day in patients with moderate hepatic impairment or in patients also being treated with a potent CYP3A4 inhibitor.

Products:

Extended-release tablets – 7.5 mg, 15 mg.

Comments:

Darifenacin has been suggested to have a selective action on the muscarinic receptors involved in bladder contraction. However, its efficacy and incidence of anticholinergic adverse events do not distinguish it from the other agents used in the treatment of overactive bladder. Most of the adverse events and precautions associated with its use are related to its anticholinergic activity. Concurrent use with another agent having anticholinergic activity (e.g., diphenhydramine [e.g., Benadryl]) may increase the severity of anticholinergic adverse events.

Because darifenacin is metabolized via two major metabolic pathways, it may interact with more medications than the other agents used in the treatment of overactive bladder. The activity of darifenacin may be significantly increased by the concurrent use of a potent CYP3A4 inhibitor (e.g., clarithromycin) and the dosage of the new drug should not exceed 7.5 mg once a day in patients treated with both agents. Darifenacin may increase the action of medications that are predominantly metabolized via CYP2D6 and which have a narrow therapeutic window (e.g., thioridazine [e.g., Mellaril], tricyclic antidepressants).

Darunavir ethanolate (Prezista – Tibotec)
Antiviral Agent
2006

New Drug Comparison Rating (NDCR) = 4 (significant advantages)

Indication:
Coadministered with ritonavir and used with other antiretroviral agents for the treatment of HIV infection in antiretroviral treatment-experienced adult patients, such as those with HIV-1 strains resistant to more than one protease inhibitor; (subsequently revised to delete restriction of use to treatment-experienced patients, and to add an indication for use in pediatric patients 6 years of age and older).

Comparable drugs:
Tipranavir (Aptivus).

Advantages:
- May be active against HIV strains that are resistant to other antiretroviral agents.
- Less risk of intracranial hemorrhaging (that is the subject of a black box warning for tipranavir).
- Less risk of clinical hepatitis and hepatic decompensation (that are the subjects of black box warnings for tipranavir).
- Dosage of ritonavir that is coadministered is lower (100 mg compared with 200 mg) and may be less likely to interact with certain medications.
- Does not need to be stored in a refrigerator.

Disadvantages:
- May be more likely to cause serious rash.
- May be more likely to interact with certain medications.

Most important risks/adverse events:
Hepatitis (liver function should be monitored before and during therapy); use is not recommended in patients with severe hepatic impairment; hyperglycemia, risk of increased bleeding in patients with hemophilia; fat redistribution; immune reconstitution syndrome; rash (treatment should be discontinued if a severe rash develops); darunavir/ritonavir inhibits the CYP3A and CYP2D6 metabolic pathways and increases the action of CYP3A and CYP2D6 substrates (contraindicated for concurrent use with oral midazolam [e.g., Versed], triazolam [e.g., Halcion], ergot-type products [e.g., dihydroergotamine], pimozide [e.g., Orap], lovastatin [e.g., Mevacor], and simvastatin [e.g., Zocor]); concurrent use with rifampin (e.g., Rifadin) and St. John's wort is also contraindicated; concurrent use may increase the activity of atorvastatin (Lipitor), phosphodiesterase type 5 inhibitors (e.g., sildenafil [Viagra]), amiodarone (e.g.,

Pacerone), bepridil (Vascor), flecainide (e.g., Tambocor), propafenone (Rythmol), quinidine, and other CYP3A and/or CYP2D6 substrates (dosage for some agents may need to be reduced); may decrease the action of methadone and it may be necessary to increase the dosage of methadone; may decrease the action of estrogens and women who are using estrogen-based oral contraceptives should be advised to use alternative or additional contraceptive measures; action may be decreased by the concurrent use of a CYP3A inducer (e.g., rifampin, St. John's wort); interactions with other antiretroviral agents may occur and require dosage adjustment of one or more agents; structure contains a sulfonamide moiety and caution must be exercised in patients with a history of sulfonamide allergy.

Most common adverse events:

Diarrhea (20%), nausea (18%), headache (15%), rash (7%).

Usual dosage:

Treatment-experienced patients - 600 mg coadministered with 100 mg of ritonavir twice a day with food; treatment-naïve patients – 800 mg with 100 mg of ritonavir once a day with food (product labeling should be consulted for dosage recommendations for pediatric patients).

Product:

Tablets – 300 mg (subsequently marketed in 75 mg, 150 mg, 400 mg, and 600 mg potencies).

Comments:

Although cross-resistance has been observed among many of the HIV protease inhibitors, clinical isolates that are resistant to the other agents in this class, including tipranavir, are often susceptible to darunavir. There apparently is only limited cross-resistance between darunavir and tipranavir.

Darunavir appears to be better tolerated than tipranavir, but may be more likely to cause serious rash.

Dasatinib (Sprycel — Bristol-Myers Squibb)
Antineoplastic Agent
2006

New Drug Comparison Rating (NDCR) = 4 (significant advantages)

Indications:

Treatment of adults with chronic, accelerated, or myeloid or lymphoid blast phase chronic myeloid leukemia (CML) with resistance or intolerance to prior therapy including imatinib; also indicated for the treatment of adults with Philadelphia chromosome-positive acute lymphoblastic leukemia (Ph+ALL) with resistance or intolerance to prior therapy.

Comparable drugs:

Imatinib (Gleevec); (another comparable drug, nilotinib [Tasigna] was subsequently marketed in late 2007).

Advantages:

- May be effective in some patients who are no longer responding to, or who can no longer tolerate, treatment with imatinib.

Disadvantages:

- Is not indicated for first-line treatment.
- Labeled indications are more limited (e.g., imatinib is also indicated for the treatment of patients with gastrointestinal stromal tumors).
- May cause QT interval prolongation.

Most important risks/adverse events:

Myelosuppression (thrombocytopenia, neutropenia, and anemia; complete blood counts should be performed weekly for the first 2 months and then at least monthly thereafter); hemorrhage; fluid retention (e.g., pleural and pericardial effusion); QT interval prolongation; may cause harm to a fetus and should not be used during pregnancy; is a substrate of CYP3A4 and action may be increased by the concurrent use of a CYP3A4 inhibitor (e.g., clarithromycin [e.g., Biaxin]), and decreased by the concurrent use of a CYP3A4 inducer (e.g., rifampin [e.g., Rifadin]); St. John's wort should not be used concurrently; absorption may be reduced by long-term suppression of gastric acid secretion and concurrent use of a proton pump inhibitor (e.g., omeprazole [e.g., Prilosec]) or a histamine H2-receptor antagonist (e.g., famotidine [e.g., Pepcid]) is not recommended; should be administered at least 2 hours apart from doses of an antacid.

Most common adverse events:

Thrombocytopenia, neutropenia, and anemia (most patients); diarrhea (49%), headache

(40%), hemorrhage (40%), musculoskeletal pain (39%), pyrexia (39%), fatigue (39%), superficial edema (36%), rash (35%), infection (34%), dyspnea (32%), cough (28%), upper respiratory tract infection (26%), abdominal pain (25%), pleural effusion (22%).

Usual dosage:

70 mg twice a day in the morning and evening (an initial dosage of 100 mg once a day for chronic phase CML and an initial dosage of 140 mg once a day for the other indications have subsequently been approved).

Products:

Tablets – 20 mg, 50 mg, 70 mg (subsequently marketed in a 100 mg potency).

Comments:

Many patients with chronic myeloid leukemia (CML) have experienced the formation of an abnormal fusion protein known as BCR-ABL that has enhanced activity as a tyrosine kinase, a class of enzymes that can cause a cascade of cellular events and uncontrolled proliferation of abnormal white blood cells. Imatinib blocks the abnormal BCR-ABL tyrosine kinase, and is often considered the first-line treatment for CML. However, some patients have experienced resistance or serious adverse events that preclude the continuation of treatment. Dasatinib is an inhibitor of multiple tyrosine kinases and, in studies in patients resistant to or intolerant of imatinib, the response rate was 45% in patients with the earliest stage of CML and ranged from 31% to 59% in patients with advanced phases of CML and Ph+ALL. Most patients who experienced a response maintained it 6 months after treatment was initiated, and the studies are ongoing. The marketing of nilotinib (Tasigna) in late 2007 provides another alternative.

Decitabine (Dacogen – Eisai)
Antineoplastic Agent
2006

New Drug Comparison Rating (NDCR) = 3 (no or minor advantages/disadvantages)

Indication:

Administered via intravenous infusion for the treatment of patients with myelodysplastic syndromes (MDS) including previously treated, untreated, de novo, and secondary MDS of all FAB (French-American-British) subtypes (refractory anemia, refractory anemia with ringed sideroblasts, refractory anemia with excess blasts, refractory anemia with excess blasts in transformation, and chronic myelomonocytic leukemia) and Intermediate-1, Intermediate-2, and High-Risk International Prognostic Scoring System groups.

Comparable drugs:

Azacitidine (Vidaza), lenalidomide (Revlimid).

Advantages:

- May provide a response in some patients who have not had an adequate response with other therapies.
- Labeled indication includes all myelodysplastic syndrome subtypes (compared with lenalidomide).
- Less risk of hepatic adverse events (compared with azacitidine).

Disadvantages:

- More likely to cause myelosuppression (compared with azacitidine).
- Must be administered intravenously (compared with azacitidine that may be administered subcutaneously or intravenously, and lenalidomide that is administered orally).

Most important risks/adverse events:

Neutropenia and thrombocytopenia (complete blood and platelet counts should be performed as needed, but at a minimum, prior to each dosing cycle); may cause harm to a fetus and should not be used during pregnancy (men should be advised not to father a child while receiving treatment, and for 2 months afterward).

Most common adverse events:

Neutropenia (90%), thrombocytopenia (89%), anemia (82%), pyrexia (53%), fatigue (48%), nausea (42%), cough (40%), petechiae (39%), constipation (35%), diarrhea (34%), hyperglycemia (33%).

Usual dosage:

Administered by continuous intravenous infusion over 3 hours; 15 mg/m^2 (as a 3-hour infusion) every 8 hours for 3 days; treatment cycle should be repeated every 6 weeks, and patients should be treated for a minimum of 4 cycles.

Product:

Vials – 50 mg; should be reconstituted with 10 mL of Sterile Water for Injection, and then further diluted with 0.9% Sodium Chloride Injection, 5% Dextrose Injection, or Lactated Ringer's Injection.

Comments:

Decitabine is an analogue of the natural nucleoside 2'-deoxycytidine, and its mechanism of action is similar to that of azacitidine, the first drug to be marketed (in 2004) for the treatment of myelodysplastic syndromes. (Earlier in 2006, lenalidomide was marketed for the treatment of a specific type of MDS associated with a deletion 5q cytogenetic abnormality). The antineoplastic effects of decitabine follow the drug's phosphorylation and direct incorporation into DNA and resulting inhibition of DNA methyltransferase, causing hypomethylation of DNA and cellular differentiation or apoptosis. In clinical studies, the overall response rate was 17% (9% complete response, 8% partial response) in patients receiving decitabine plus supportive care (transfusions, antibiotics, and hematopoietic growth factors), and 0% among those receiving supportive care alone. Benefit from the use of decitabine was observed in an additional 13% of patients who experienced hematologic improvement but did not meet the criteria for partial response or better compared with 7% of patients in the supportive care group. In patients with a complete or partial response, the median time to response was 93 days and the median duration of response was 288 days. Decitabine and azacitidine have not been directly compared in clinical studies.

Deferasirox (Exjade – Novartis)
Iron Chelator
2005

New Drug Comparison Rating (NDCR) = 4 (significant advantages)

Indication:

Treatment of chronic iron overload due to blood transfusions (transfusional hemosiderosis) in patients 2 years of age and older.

Comparable drugs:

Deferoxamine (Desferal).

Advantages:

• Administered orally.

Disadvantages:

• Higher incidence of increases in serum creatinine concentrations.
• Higher incidence of hepatic abnormalities (e.g., increases in serum aminotransferases).
• Available only through a restricted distribution program.

Most important risks/adverse events:

Acute renal failure (serum creatinine concentrations should be monitored at monthly intervals); cytopenias (e.g., agranulocytosis, neutropenia, thrombocytopenia; blood counts should be monitored at regular intervals); hepatic failure (liver function tests should be monitored every two weeks during the first month and monthly thereafter); gastrointestinal irritation (ulcer, bleeding; use caution in patients also taking other drugs with an ulcerogenic or hemorrhagic potential); auditory and ocular disturbances (testing is recommended on an annual basis); should not be taken with an aluminum-containing antacid.

Most common adverse events:

Elevations of serum creatinine concentrations (38%), pyrexia (19%), headache (16%), cough (14%), abdominal pain (14%), diarrhea (12%), nausea (11%), vomiting (10%), rash (8%).

Usual dosage:

20 mg/kg once a day, administered on an empty stomach at least 30 minutes before food, preferably at the same time each day; serum ferritin concentrations should be monitored every month and the dosage should be adjusted, if necessary, every 3 to 6 months based on serum ferritin trends; dosage should not exceed 30 mg/kg/day (has

been subsequently revised to 40 mg/kg/day; dosage may be increased when a potent UGT inducer [e.g., phenytoin, rifampin] is used concurrently).

Products:

Tablets (for oral suspension) – 125 mg, 250 mg, 500 mg; tablets should be completely dispersed by stirring in water, orange juice, or apple juice until a fine suspension is obtained; tablets should not be swallowed whole or chewed.

Comments:

Iron overload is a potentially life-threatening consequence of frequent blood transfusions used in the treatment of rare, chronic blood disorders including thalassemia and sickle cell disease, as well as in other rare anemias and myelodysplastic syndromes. Iron overload may become evident following transfusion of approximately 20 units of blood and, if not treated, excess iron may cause damage to the heart, liver, and endocrine glands.

Iron chelation therapy has been used in the treatment of transfusion-related iron overload and, by binding to iron, the chelating agent helps remove it via the urine and/or feces. Deferoxamine has been the standard therapy, but it must be administered parenterally via prolonged infusions (e.g., 8 to 12 hours) and many patients have interrupted or stopped treatment. Deferasirox is the first orally effective chelating agent that is selective for iron (as ferric iron), and it has been demonstrated to be effective in reducing liver iron concentrations in patients receiving transfusions on an ongoing basis.

Dose-dependent increases in serum creatinine concentrations have occurred at a greater frequency (38%) than in deferoxamine-treated patients (15%), although most of the creatinine elevations remained in the normal range. Renal function and liver function should be monitored at least monthly.

Degarelix acetate (Firmagon – Ferring)
Antineoplastic Agent
2009

New Drug Comparison Rating (NDCR) = 4 (significant advantages)

Indication:
Administered subcutaneously for the treatment of patients with advanced prostate cancer.

Comparable drugs:
Leuprolide (e.g., Lupron, Eligard), goserelin (Zoladex), triptorelin (Trelstar); (The previously marketed drug to which degarelix is most similar is abarelix [Plenaxis] that was marketed in 2004; however, this drug is no longer marketed in the United States and the comparisons noted below are with leuprolide, goserelin, and triptorelin).

Advantages:
- Unique mechanism of action in treating prostate cancer (gonadotropin-releasing hormone [GnRH] receptor antagonist).
- Does not cause an increase in testosterone concentrations when treatment is initiated.
- May be used in some patients for whom other therapies are not appropriate.

Disadvantages:
- Labeled indications are more limited (compared with leuprolide that is also indicated for the treatment of endometriosis, uterine leiomyomata [fibroids], and central precocious puberty, and goserelin that is also indicated for the treatment of advanced breast cancer, endometriosis, and endometrial thinning).
- More likely to cause injection site reactions.
- Fewer formulation options (e.g., the comparable drugs are available in formulations that provide a longer duration of action [e.g., 3 months/84 days]).

Most important risks/adverse events:
If used off-label in women, may cause harm to a fetus and is contraindicated in women who are or may become pregnant (Pregnancy Category X); QT interval prolongation (caution must be exercised in patients at risk [e.g., those with electrolyte abnormalities, concurrent use of other medications with this risk]); may alter the results of diagnostic tests of the pituitary gonadotropic and gonadal functions.

Most common adverse events:
Injection site reactions (35%), hot flashes (26%), increased weight (9%), hypertension (6%), back pain (6%), arthralgia (5%), urinary tract infections (5%), chills (5%), constipation (5%), increases in serum transaminases and gamma-glutamyltransferase (10%).

Usual dosage:

240 mg initially administered as two deep subcutaneous injections of 120 mg at a concentration of 40 mg/mL; maintenance dosage is 80 mg every 28 days administered as one subcutaneous injection at a concentration of 20 mg/mL; injections should be administered in the abdominal area.

Products:

Vials – 80 mg, 120 mg; reconstitution (with Sterile Water for Injection) and administration procedures should be performed while keeping the vials vertical, and by gently swirling the vials when the diluent is added; Treatment Initiation pack contains two vials (each containing 120 mg) for two subcutaneous injections, and Treatment Maintenance pack contains one vial with 80 mg of the drug.

Comments:

Gonadotropin-releasing hormone (GnRH) agonists (leuprolide, goserelin, triptorelin) have been effective in the treatment of many patients with prostate cancer. However, these agents cause an initial surge/increase in testosterone concentrations before the substantial reduction in its concentration occurs, and some patients are not able to tolerate the initial testosterone surge. Degarelix acts as a GnRH receptor antagonist that binds to the pituitary GnRH receptors, thereby reducing the release of gonadotropins and consequently testosterone. Its properties are most similar to those of abarelix that is no longer marketed in the United States because of the risk of serious allergic reactions and other restrictions to its use. The effectiveness of degarelix was demonstrated in clinical studies in which it was compared with leuprolide (7.5 mg intramuscularly once a month). The primary endpoint was the reduction of serum testosterone to castration concentrations, and was attained in more than 95% of the patients with each drug. The drug forms a depot at the injection site from which it is slowly released into the circulation.

Desvenlafaxine succinate (Pristiq – Wyeth)
Antidepressant
2008

New Drug Comparison Rating (NDCR) = 3 (no or minor advantages/disadvantages)

Indication:
Treatment of patients with major depressive disorder.

Comparable drug:
Venlafaxine extended-release capsules (Effexor XR).

Advantages:
- Dosage titration usually not necessary.
- Less risk of interactions with CYP2D6 inducers or inhibitors.
- Dosage reduction is not necessary in patients with hepatic impairment.

Disadvantages:
- Has not been directly compared with venlafaxine in clinical studies.
- Fewer labeled indications (venlafaxine extended-release also has indications for generalized anxiety disorder, panic disorder, and social anxiety disorder).

Most important risks/adverse events:
Risk of suicidal thinking and behavior in children, adolescents, and young adults (boxed warning [is not indicated for use in pediatric patients]); serotonin syndrome (risk is greater in patients who are also treated with other drugs that may affect serotonergic systems [e.g., selective serotonin reuptake inhibitors (SSRIs), serotonin and norepinephrine reuptake inhibitors (SNRIs), triptans], or drugs that impair metabolism of serotonin [monoamine oxidase inhibitors (MAOIs)]); activation of mania/hypomania; seizures; hyponatremia; interstitial lung disease and eosinophilic pneumonia; elevated blood pressure (pre-existing hypertension should be controlled before initiating treatment; blood pressure should be regularly monitored); elevated cholesterol and triglyceride concentrations; mydriasis (patients with increased intraocular pressure should be monitored); bleeding events (e.g., ecchymosis, epistaxis; risk is increased by the concurrent use of anticoagulants, aspirin, and nonsteroidal anti-inflammatory drugs); Pregnancy Category C (risk of complications has been reported to be increased if used during the third trimester); contraindicated in patients being treated with an MAOI or within 14 days of discontinuing treatment with an MAOI; treatment with an MAOI should not be initiated for at least 7 days following discontinuation of desvenlafaxine; caution should be exercised when used concurrently with other central nervous system-active drugs; patients should be advised to avoid consuming alcoholic beverages; action may be increased by the concurrent use of a

potent CYP3A4 inhibitor (e.g., clarithromycin [e.g., Biaxin]); concurrent use with tryptophan supplements should be avoided.

Most common adverse events:

Nausea (22%), dizziness (13%), dry mouth (11%), hyperhidrosis (10%), constipation (9%), insomnia (9%), fatigue (7%), decreased appetite (5%), somnolence (4%), male sexual function disorders (e.g., decreased libido; 4%).

Usual dosage:

50 mg once a day; patients should be advised that the tablets should be swallowed whole and that the tablet should not be divided, crushed, chewed, or dissolved; patients should also be informed that they may observe the inert matrix tablet in the stool but that the active medication has already been absorbed; a dosage higher than 100 mg once a day should not be exceeded in patients with hepatic impairment; a dosage of 50 mg once a day is recommended in patients with moderate renal impairment, and a dosage of 50 mg every other day is recommended in patients with severe renal impairment (creatinine clearance less than 30 mL/minute); when treatment is to be discontinued, the dosage should be gradually reduced by administering 50 mg of the drug less frequently rather than abruptly stopping therapy.

Product:

Extended-release tablets – 50 mg, 100 mg.

Comments:

Desvenlafaxine is the major active metabolite of venlafaxine that is pharmacologically approximately equiactive and equipotent to its parent compound. Like venlafaxine, as well as duloxetine (Cymbalta), desvenlafaxine is a serotonin and norepinephrine reuptake inhibitor. The effectiveness of desvenlafaxine in the treatment of patients with major depressive disorder has been demonstrated in four 8-week, placebo-controlled studies in adult patients. However, it has not been directly compared with venlafaxine in clinical studies and there is no reason to consider it to be more effective than venlafaxine. Venlafaxine also has labeled indications for the treatment of generalized anxiety, social anxiety, and panic disorders. However, these are not labeled indications for desvenlafaxine at the present time, although the new agent is being studied for the treatment of other conditions.

The drug-related problems associated with the use of desvenlafaxine are generally similar to those for venlafaxine and duloxetine, as well as the selective serotonin reuptake inhibitors (SSRIs; e.g., fluoxetine [e.g., Prozac]). The CYP2D6 metabolic pathway is the most important pathway through which venlafaxine is converted to desvenlafaxine. However, this pathway is not involved in the metabolism of desvenlafaxine and it is not likely to interact with other medications that are inhibitors or inducers of the CYP2D6 pathway.

Difluprednate (Durezol – Sirion)
Ophthalmic Corticosteroid
2008

New Drug Comparison Rating (NDCR) = 4 (significant advantages)

Indication:
For ophthalmic use for the treatment of inflammation and pain associated with ocular surgery.

Comparable drugs:
Ophthalmic corticosteroids used in conjunction with ocular surgery; loteprednol etabonate (Lotemax), rimexolone (Vexol).

Advantages:
- First ophthalmic corticosteroid to be demonstrated to be effective in the treatment of pain associated with ocular surgery (other agents are indicated only for the treatment of inflammation).
- Emulsion formulation may provide more uniform drug delivery and enhance intraocular penetration (loteprednol and rimexolone are supplied in ophthalmic suspension formulations).

Disadvantages:
- Has not been directly compared in clinical studies with other ophthalmic corticosteroids in patients having ocular surgery.
- Labeled indications are more limited (loteprednol and rimexolone are also indicated for ophthalmic inflammatory conditions not associated with surgery, and loteprednol is also indicated [in a lower-potency formulation (Alrex)] for seasonal allergic conjunctivitis).

Most important risks/adverse events:
Contraindicated in patients with viral diseases of the cornea and conjunctiva such as epithelial herpes simplex keratitis, vaccinia, and varicella, and also in mycobacterial infection of the eye and fungal diseases of ocular structures [fungal invasion should be considered in patients who experience persistent corneal ulceration]); increased risk of secondary ocular infections; increased intraocular pressure (IOP) that could result in glaucoma with damage to the optic nerve, and defects in visual acuity and fields of vision (IOP should be monitored if used for 10 days or longer); posterior subcapsular cataract formation; may delay healing.

Most common adverse events (each at an incidence of 5% - 15%):

Corneal edema, ciliary and conjunctival hyperemia, eye pain, photophobia, posterior capsule opacification, anterior chamber cells, anterior chamber flare, conjunctival edema, blepharitis.

Usual dosage:

One drop into the conjunctival sac of the affected eye(s) 4 times daily beginning 24 hours after surgery and continuing throughout the first 2 weeks of the postoperative period, followed by 2 times daily for a week and then a taper based on the response.

Product:

Ophthalmic emulsion – 0.05%.

Comments:

Ophthalmic surgeries (e.g., cataract surgery) frequently result in postoperative inflammation which, if left untreated, may interfere with a patient's visual rehabilitation and result in complications. Ophthalmic formulations of corticosteroids and nonsteroidal anti-inflammatory drugs (NSAIDs; e.g., nepafenac [Nevanac]) are frequently used in the treatment of inflammation following eye surgery. Difluprednate is the ninth corticosteroid on the market in ophthalmic formulations for the treatment of ocular inflammatory conditions. Loteprednol and rimexolone are the only other corticosteroids used in conjunction with ocular surgery; these agents are indicated for inflammation associated with ocular surgery whereas difluprednate is the first ophthalmic corticosteroid to also be demonstrated to be effective for the treatment of postoperative pain. The effectiveness of difluprednate has been demonstrated in two placebo (vehicle)-controlled studies in which relief of pain was reported 15 days following surgery in 63% of patients treated with the new drug, compared with 35% of those receiving placebo.

The emulsion formulation of difluprednate was developed to provide uniform drug delivery and enhance intraocular penetration compared to an ophthalmic suspension of the drug. However, the new drug has not been directly compared with the suspension formulations of loteprednol and rimexolone. The emulsion does not have to be shaken prior to administration. It should be protected from light.

Doripenem (Doribax – Ortho-McNeil)
Antibiotic
2007

New Drug Comparison Rating (NDCR) = 3 (no or minor advantages/disadvantages)

Indications:
Administered via intravenous infusion for the treatment of complicated intra-abdominal infections, and complicated urinary tract infections, including pyelonephritis caused by susceptible organisms.

Comparable drugs:
Imipenem/cilastatin (Primaxin), meropenem (Merrem IV), ertapenem (Invanz).

Advantages:
- Does not require inclusion of cilastatin for optimum activity (compared with imipenem).
- More active against Pseudomonas aeruginosa and Acinetobacter (compared with ertapenem).

Disadvantages:
- Fewer labeled indications.
- Shorter duration of action (compared with ertapenem that may be administered once a day in most patients).
- Not indicated for use in pediatric patients.
- Fewer options for parenteral administration (compared with imipenem and ertapenem that may be administered intramuscularly as well as intravenously).

Most important risks/adverse events:
Hypersensitivity reactions (contraindicated in patients who are hypersensitive to other carbapenems [e.g., imipenem] and in patients who have demonstrated anaphylactic reactions to other beta-lactam antibiotics [e.g., penicillins, cephalosporins]); dosage should be reduced in patients with renal impairment; may reduce serum concentrations and activity of valproic acid (e.g., Depakene).

Most common adverse events (incidence as reported in patients with intra-abdominal infections):
Nausea (12%), diarrhea (11%), anemia (10%), phlebitis (8%), rash (5%), headache (4%).

Usual dosage:

Administered via intravenous infusion over one hour; 500 mg every 8 hours; in patients with a creatinine clearance between 30 and 50 mL/minute, dosage should be reduced to 250 mg every 8 hours; in patients with a creatinine clearance greater than 10 and less than 30 mL/minute, dosage should be reduced to 250 mg every 12 hours.

Product:

Vials – 500 mg.

Comments:

Doripenem is the fourth carbapenem beta-lactam antibiotic to be marketed in the United States, joining imipenem, meropenem, and ertapenem. The four agents are administered parenterally and have a broad spectrum of action that includes many gram-positive and gram-negative aerobic and anaerobic bacteria. Doripenem is primarily active against gram-negative bacteria including Pseudomonas aeruginosa and Acinetobacter baumannii, and is effective as a single agent in the infections caused by the bacteria identified in its labeled indications. In the clinical trials, doripenem was non-inferior to meropenem in the treatment of patients with complicated intra-abdominal infections, and non-inferior to levofloxacin (Levaquin) in patients with complicated urinary tract infections. The broad spectrum of action of the carbapenems may result in their being effective as single agents in the treatment of mixed infections that might otherwise have required the use of at least two antibiotics.

Dronedarone hydrochloride (Multaq – Sanofi-Aventis)
Antiarrhythmic Agent
2009

New Drug Comparison Rating (NDCR) = 4 (significant advantages)

Indication:

To reduce the risk of cardiovascular hospitalization in patients with paroxysmal or persistent atrial fibrillation (AF) or atrial flutter (AFL), with a recent episode of AF/AFL and associated cardiovascular risk factors (i.e., age>70, hypertension, diabetes, prior cerebrovascular accident, left atrial diameter of 50 mm or greater, or left ventricular ejection fraction <40%), who are in sinus rhythm or who will be cardioverted.

Comparable drug:

Amiodarone (e.g., Cordarone).

Advantages:

- Has a labeled indication for use in patients with atrial fibrillation and atrial flutter (whereas the labeled indications for amiodarone are for the treatment of ventricular arrhythmias).
- Less likely to cause pulmonary, thyroid, hepatic, or ocular adverse events.
- Has not been reported to cause blue-gray discoloration of skin.
- Is not likely to interact with warfarin.
- May be used in patients who are hypersensitive to iodine (whereas amiodarone is contraindicated because iodine is a component of its structure).
- Dosage adjustment is not necessary.

Disadvantages:

- Is less effective (based on the results of a study that directly compared the two drugs).
- Is not indicated for the treatment of ventricular arrhythmias.
- Increased risk of mortality in patients with severe heart failure (use is contraindicated).
- Is in Pregnancy Category X and is contraindicated during pregnancy (whereas amiodarone is in Pregnancy Category D).
- Has more contraindications.
- Is administered more frequently (twice a day whereas amiodarone may often be administered once a day).

Most important risks/adverse events:

Increased risk of mortality in patients with severe heart failure (boxed warning) and use is contraindicated in patients with NYHA Class IV heart failure or NYHA Class II-III heart failure with a recent decompensation requiring hospitalization or a referral to a specialized heart failure clinic; contraindicated in patients with second- or third-degree atrioventricular block or sick sinus syndrome (except when used in conjunction with a functioning pacemaker), and in patients with bradycardia <50 bpm; may prolong the QT interval (concurrent use of other agents that prolong the QT interval is contraindicated, as is use in patients with a QTcBazett interval of 500 ms or greater; potassium and magnesium concentrations should be maintained in the normal range);

action is increased by the concomitant use of a strong CYP3A inhibitor (e.g., clarithromycin) and concurrent use is contraindicated; is contraindicated in patients with severe hepatic impairment; may cause fetal harm (Pregnancy Category X) and use is contraindicated during pregnancy (women of childbearing potential should use effective contraception) and in nursing mothers; may cause a small increase in serum creatinine concentrations; action may be increased by CYP3A inhibitors (e.g., use of grapefruit juice should be avoided), and decreased by CYP3A inducers (e.g., rifampin, St. John's wort; concurrent use should be avoided); may increase the action of CYP3A substrates (e.g., simvastatin) and CYP2D6 substrates (e.g., fluoxetine); concurrent use with digoxin may increase the action of both agents (if digoxin treatment is continued, the dosage should be reduced by one-half); when a beta-blocker (e.g., metoprolol) or calcium channel blocker (e.g., diltiazem, verapamil) is to be used in a patient treated with dronedarone, they should be used initially in a low dosage.

Most common adverse events:

Diarrhea (8%), asthenia (7%), nausea (5%), dermatologic effects (5% – e.g., rash, pruritus), abdominal pain (4%), bradycardia (3%).

Usual dosage:

400 mg twice a day with the morning and evening meals.

Product:

Film-coated tablets – 400 mg.

Comments:

Dronedarone is a benzofuran antiarrhythmic agent that has structural and pharmacological properties that are most similar to those of amiodarone. It exhibits electrophysiologic effects that include characteristics of all four Vaughan-Williams classes of antiarrhythmic agents. It is indicated to reduce the risk of cardiovascular hospitalization in patients with paroxysmal or persistent atrial fibrillation or atrial flutter (see indication above). The labeled indications for amiodarone are the treatment of recurrent ventricular fibrillation and recurrent hemodynamically unstable ventricular tachycardia, although it is often used "off-label" for the treatment of patients with atrial arrhythmias. The effectiveness of dronedarone was demonstrated in studies in which it reduced the combined endpoint of cardiovascular hospitalization or death from any cause by 24% when compared to placebo. The benefit of the drug was entirely attributable to its reduction of cardiovascular hospitalization. In one study that included patients with severe heart failure, the trial was terminated because of a higher mortality rate (8%) in patients treated with dronedarone compared with a rate of 4% in those receiving placebo. In a study in which it was directly compared with amiodarone, dronedarone was considered less effective in reducing recurrences of atrial fibrillation but was better tolerated, as reflected by fewer discontinuations of treatment because of the occurrence of adverse events.

Dronedarone is less likely than amiodarone to cause pulmonary, thyroid, hepatic, and ocular adverse events, and skin discoloration. However, it is more likely to cause serious complications in patients with severe heart failure and its use is, therefore, contraindicated in such patients. Both drugs interact with numerous other medications. Dronedarone undergoes extensive presystemic first-pass metabolism and its absolute bioavailability is 4% when it is administered apart from food. It should be administered twice a day with the morning and evening meals.

Ecamsule (Anthelios SX [with avobenzone and octocrylene] – LaRoche-Posay)
Sunscreen
2006

New Drug Comparison Rating (NDCR) = 4 (significant advantages)

Indications:
Applied topically for the prevention of sunburn and protection from UVA and UVB rays (used as a daily skin moisturizing product); (subsequently approved in a second formulation that also contains titanium dioxide and that is used as a sunscreen cream for the face and body).

Comparable drugs:
Octocrylene, avobenzone.

Advantages:
- More protective against short UVA rays.
- Does not degrade when exposed to the sun for long periods of time.

Disadvantages:
- Less protective than octocrylene against UVB rays.
- Less protective than avobenzone against longer UVA rays.

Most important risks/adverse events:
None.

Most common adverse events:
Acne, dermatitis, eczema, itching, skin discomfort (these events occur infrequently).

Usual dosage:
For use as a daily moisturizing product, apply evenly to the skin and reapply as needed or after towel drying, swimming, or perspiring.

Products:
Moisturizing cream (Anthelios SX) – 2% ecamsule, 2% avobenzone, 10% octocrylene (SPF 15); sunscreen cream (Anthelios 20; Capital Soleil 20) – 2% ecamsule, 2% avobenzone, 10% octocrylene, 2% titanium dioxide (SPF 20); sunscreen cream (Anthelios 40) – 3% ecamsule, 2% avobenzone, 10% octocrylene, 5% titanium dioxide (SPF 40); products are available without a prescription.

Comments:

The ultraviolet spectrum comprises three major bands: UVA, UVB, and UVC. The wavelength of UVC ranges from 200 to 290 nm but little of this radiation reaches the earth. The wavelength of the UVB band is 290 to 320 nm. The high energy of this radiation is primarily concentrated in the epidermal level and is most often associated with the occurrence of acute erythema (sunburn), although it also plays a role in the occurrence of certain skin cancers and chronic dermatoses. Most sunscreen products identify a sun protection factor (SPF) that represents the level of protection against UVB. The wavelength of the UVA band is from 320 to 400 nm. It is further classified as short (320-340 nm) and long (340-400 nm) UVA radiation. Unlike UVB, UVA radiation is present every day throughout the year.

Ecamsule is a sunscreen that has been available in other countries under the designation Mexoryl SX. It is not available as a single agent in the United States. It is highly protective against short UVA rays and was initially approved for nonprescription use as part of a combination formulation that also contains avobenzone, which protects against the longer UVA rays, and octocrylene, which protects against UVB rays. Used in combination, the three agents provide broad-spectrum sun protection and this formulation has been used as a daily moisturizing product. Subsequently, additional formulations that also contain a fourth sunscreen, titanium dioxide, have been approved for use as "beach" products.

Eculizumab (Soliris – Alexion)
Agent for Paroxysmal Nocturnal Hemoglobinuria
2007

New Drug Comparison Rating (NDCR) = 5 (important advance)

Indication:
Administered via intravenous infusion for the treatment of patients with paroxysmal nocturnal hemoglobinuria (PNH) to reduce hemolysis.

Comparable drugs:
None.

Advantages:
- First drug to be approved for the treatment of PNH.
- Patients needed fewer blood transfusions and reported improved quality of life.

Disadvantages/Limitations:
- Risk of meningococcal infection (vaccination is required).
- Must be administered parenterally.
- Available only through a restricted distribution program.

Most important risks/adverse events:
Risk of meningococcal infection (boxed warning; patients should be vaccinated with a meningococcal vaccine at least 2 weeks prior to receiving the first dose, and should be revaccinated according to current guidelines; patients should be monitored for early signs of meningococcal infection); risk of other infections; if therapy is discontinued, patients should be monitored for signs and symptoms of intravascular hemolysis, including evaluation of serum lactate dehydrogenase (LDH) concentrations.

Most common adverse events:
Headache (44%), nasopharyngitis (23%), back pain (19%), nausea (16%), fatigue (12%).

Usual dosage:
Administered via a 35-minute intravenous infusion via gravity feed, a syringe-type pump, or an infusion pump; 600 mg every 7 days for the first 4 weeks, followed by 900 mg for the fifth dose 7 days later, and then 900 mg every 14 days thereafter; patients should be monitored for at least 1 hour after completion of an infusion for signs or symptoms of an infusion reaction.

Product:

Vials – 300 mg (30 mL of a 10 mg/mL solution; should be stored in a refrigerator); solution should be diluted to a final admixture concentration of 5 mg/mL.

Comments:

Paroxysmal nocturnal hemoglobinuria (PNH) is a rare blood disorder that can lead to disability and premature death. Patients with PNH have a genetic mutation that leads to the development of abnormal red blood cells that are deficient in terminal complement inhibitors. This deficiency makes the red blood cells vulnerable to terminal complement-mediated destruction and intravascular hemolysis. The loss of red blood cells results in anemia, hemoglobinuria, dark urine, fatigue, debilitating weakness, shortness of breath, and blood clots, as well as an increased risk of stroke and heart attacks. Periodic blood transfusions and immunosuppressive therapy have been of benefit for some patients.

Eculizumab is a recombinant humanized monoclonal antibody that specifically binds to the complement protein C5 and inhibits terminal complement-mediated intravascular hemolysis in patients with PNH. It is the first drug to be approved for the treatment of PNH. It does not cure PNH but reduces the destruction of PNH red blood cells and the occurrence of related complications. In a placebo-controlled study, one-half of the patients receiving the drug experienced stabilization of hemoglobin concentrations, compared with none of the patients receiving placebo. Eculizumab-treated patients also needed significantly fewer blood transfusions and reported less fatigue and improved quality of life.

Because it inhibits the immune system, eculizumab increases the risk of infection. Of particular concern is the potential for meningococcal infections (i.e., septicemia, meningitis) and the drug is contraindicated in patients with unresolved Neisseria meningitidis infection and in patients who are not currently vaccinated against N. meningitidis.

Eltrombopag olamine (Promacta – GlaxoSmithKline)
Agent for Immune Thrombocytopenic Purpura
2008

New Drug Comparison Rating (NDCR) = 4 (significant advantages)

Indication:

Treatment of thrombocytopenia in patients with chronic immune (idiopathic) thrombocytopenic purpura (ITP) who have had an insufficient response to corticosteroids, immunoglobulins, or splenectomy; should be used only in patients with ITP whose degree of thrombocytopenia and clinical condition increase the risk of bleeding; it should not be used in an attempt to normalize platelet counts.

Comparable drugs:

Romiplostim (Nplate).

Advantages:

- Is administered orally (romiplostim is administered subcutaneously).
- Is not associated with the development of neutralizing antibodies.

Disadvantages:

- May cause hepatotoxicity.
- Has been associated with development or worsening of cataracts.
- More likely to interact with other medications.
- Available only through a restricted distribution program.

Most important risks/adverse events:

May cause hepatotoxicity (boxed warning; serum ALT, AST, and bilirubin should be measured prior to initiating treatment, every two weeks during the dosage adjustment phase, and monthly following the establishment of a stable dosage; must be used with caution in patients with hepatic impairment); increases the risk of reticulin deposition in the bone marrow (that may increase the risk of bone marrow fibrosis); excessive doses may increase platelet count to a level that produces thrombotic/thromboembolic complications; may increase the risk for hematological malignancies; discontinuation of treatment may result in thrombocytopenia that is worse than that which was present prior to treatment; has been associated with the development or worsening of cataracts; may cause fetal harm – Pregnancy Category C (women who are pregnant should be enrolled in a pregnancy registry); inhibits organic anion transporting polypeptide OATP1B1 and may increase the action of medications (e.g., rosuvastatin [Crestor]) that are substrates for this metabolic pathway; absorption and activity may be significantly reduced by polyvalent cations and should not be administered within 4 hours of any medication or product containing polyvalent cations (e.g., antacids, dairy products, mineral supplements).

Most common adverse events:

Nausea (6%), vomiting (4%), menorrhagia (4%), myalgia (3%), paresthesia (3%), cataract (3%).

Usual dosage:

Initially, 50 mg once a day on an empty stomach (1 hour before or 2 hours after a meal); in patients of East Asian ancestry (i.e., Chinese, Japanese, Korean, Taiwanese) and in those with modest or severe hepatic impairment, the recommended initial dosage is 25 mg once a day; the dosage is subsequently adjusted to achieve and maintain a platelet count of at least 50×10^9/Liter to reduce the risk for bleeding; maximum recommended daily dose is 75 mg.

Products:

Tablets – 25 mg, 50 mg.

Comments:

Eltrombopag is the second drug to be approved for the treatment of thrombocytopenia in patients with chronic ITP, following by several months the approval of romiplostim. It is a small molecule thrombopoietin (TPO) receptor agonist that is effective following oral administration. By interacting with the transmembrane domain of TPO receptors, eltrombopag increases platelet production. Eltrombopag was evaluated in two placebo-controlled studies in which the target platelet count response was attained in 59% and 70% of patients, compared with 16% and 11%, respectively, of those receiving placebo. In addition to the drug interactions noted above, eltrombopag is a substrate for CYP1A2, CYP2C8, UGT1A1, and UGT1A3, and its action may be altered by inhibitors or inducers of these pathways.

Entecavir (Baraclude – Bristol-Myers Squibb)
Antiviral Agent
2005

New Drug Comparison Rating (NDCR) = 4 (significant advantages)

Indication:

Treatment of chronic hepatitis B virus (HBV) infection in adults with evidence of active viral replication and either evidence of persistent elevations in serum aminotransferases (ALT or AST) or histologically active disease.

Comparable drugs:

Adefovir dipivoxil (Hepsera), lamivudine (Epivir-HBV); (subsequent to the marketing of entecavir, telbivudine [Tyzeka] has also been marketed for the treatment of chronic HBV infection, and the indications for tenofovir [Viread] have been expanded to include chronic HBV infection).

Advantages:

• May be effective in patients who are refractory to lamivudine.
• Does not appear to be active against HIV and, in patients who are co-infected with HBV and HIV, is not likely to reduce the efficacy of the antiviral agents against HIV.

Disadvantages:

• Not indicated in patients less than 16 years of age (compared with lamivudine that is indicated for use in children as young as 2 years of age).

Most important risks/adverse events:

Lactic acidosis and severe hepatomegaly with steatosis (boxed warning); severe acute exacerbations of hepatitis upon discontinuation of treatment (boxed warning); potential for the development of resistance to HIV nucleoside reverse transcriptase inhibitors if entecavir is used to treat chronic HBV infection in patients with HIV infection that is not being treated (boxed warning; treatment with entecavir is not recommended in HIV/HBV co-infected patients who are not also receiving highly active antiretroviral therapy).

Most common adverse events:

Headache (4%), fatigue (3%).

Usual dosage:

0.5 mg once a day in nucleoside-treatment-naïve patients; 1 mg once a day in patients with a history of hepatitis B viremia while being treated with lamivudine or known lamivudine resistance mutations; dosage should be reduced in patients with impaired renal function.

Products:

Tablets – 0.5 mg, 1 mg; oral solution – 0.05 mg/mL.

Comments:

Entecavir is a guanosine nucleoside analogue that is phosphorylated to its triphosphate form that is active against HBV polymerase (reverse transcriptase). In studies in which it was compared with lamivudine, it provided better results in attaining the primary efficacy endpoint of histologic improvement, and on the secondary efficacy measures of reduction of viral load and ALT normalization. It was also evaluated in lamivudine-refractory patients, and many patients experienced improvement with its use.

Since the time entecavir was marketed in 2005, telbivudine has been marketed (2006) for the treatment of chronic HBV infection and the indications for tenofovir [Viread] have been expanded (2008) to include chronic HBV infection.

Eszopiclone (Lunesta –Sepracor)
Hypnotic
2005

New Drug Comparison Rating (NDCR) = 3 (no or minor advantages/disadvantages)

Indication:
Treatment of insomnia.

Comparable drugs:
Zaleplon (Sonata), zolpidem (Ambien), temazepam (e.g., Restoril); (The controlled-release formulation of zolpidem [Ambien CR] was marketed after the marketing of eszopiclone.).

Advantages:
- Labeling does not include a limit with respect to duration of use.
- Long duration of action may be of benefit with respect to maintaining sleep and decreasing early-morning awakening.

Disadvantages:
- Long duration of action may increase the likelihood of daytime sedation.
- Unpleasant taste is a common adverse event.
- Extensively metabolized via the CYP3A4 pathway and is more likely to interact with other medications.
- Pregnancy Category C (compared with zolpidem which is in category B).

Most important risks/adverse events:
Potential for an excessive central nervous system depressant effect; consumption of alcoholic beverages should be avoided; potential for misuse/abuse (is a controlled substance classified in Schedule IV); is extensively metabolized via the CYP3A4 pathway and action may be significantly increased by the concurrent use of a potent CYP3A4 inhibitor (e.g., clarithromycin [e.g., Biaxin]).

Most common adverse events:
Headache (21%), unpleasant taste (17%), somnolence (10%), dizziness (5%), dry mouth (5%)—incidences reported are with a dosage of 2 mg at bedtime and are higher for most of these events with a dosage of 3 mg at bedtime.

Usual dosage:
2 mg immediately before bedtime; if the primary complaint is difficulty staying asleep, the dosage may be initiated at or raised to 3 mg at bedtime (2 mg in elderly patients); a starting dosage of 1 mg at bedtime is recommended for elderly patients whose primary

complaint is difficulty in falling asleep; in patients with severe hepatic impairment or who are being treated concurrently with a potent CYP3A4 inhibitor, the recommended starting dosage is 1 mg at bedtime.

Products:

Tablets – 1 mg, 2 mg, 3 mg.

Comments:

Eszopiclone is the active S-isomer of zopiclone, a racemic mixture that has been investigated as a hypnotic but is not marketed in the United States. The properties of eszopiclone are most similar to those of zolpidem. Neither agent is a benzodiazepine (e.g., temazepam) but they are believed to act at gamma aminobutyric acid (GABA) receptors at which the benzodiazepines interact.

Both eszopiclone and zolpidem have a rapid onset of action but eszopiclone has a longer duration of action. Eszopiclone has been demonstrated to be effective in the treatment of insomnia characterized by difficulty in falling asleep and difficulty in maintaining sleep, whereas the effectiveness of zolpidem has been primarily established in patients with difficulty in falling asleep. (A controlled-release formulation of zolpidem [Ambien CR] was marketed after eszopiclone reached the market, and is also effective in maintaining sleep.) Although the longer duration of action of eszopiclone is an advantage in maintaining sleep and decreasing early-morning awakening, it is also a disadvantage because of the greater likelihood of daytime sedation. It is recommended that eszopiclone not be used in patients who are not able to get at least 8 hours of sleep before they must be active again.

The use of many hypnotics has been studied over a period of 28 to 35 days and their labeling recommends that their use be limited to that duration of time. Studies of eszopiclone were continued over a period of 6 months without evidence of important problems when treatment was discontinued.

Etravirine (Intelence – Tibotec)
Antiviral Agent
2008

New Drug Comparison Rating (NDCR) = 4 (significant advantages)

Indication:

In combination with other antiretroviral agents for the treatment of HIV-1 infection in treatment-experienced adult patients, who have evidence of viral replication and HIV-1 strains resistant to a non-nucleoside reverse transcriptase inhibitor (NNRTI) and other antiretroviral agents.

Comparable drugs:

Non-nucleoside reverse transcriptase inhibitors (NNRTIs): Delavirdine (Rescriptor), efavirenz (Sustiva), nevirapine (Viramune).

Advantages:

- Is effective in some patients who have become resistant to other antiretroviral regimens.
- Not likely to cause hepatic adverse events (compared with nevirapine that has a boxed warning in its labeling regarding this risk).
- Not likely to cause central nervous system and psychiatric adverse events (compared with efavirenz).
- May have less risk when used during pregnancy (is in Pregnancy Category B; compared with delavirdine that is in Category C and efavirenz that is in Category D).
- Certain drug interactions may be of lesser clinical importance (e.g., compared with efavirenz for which certain interacting drugs are identified as being contraindicated).
- Is administered less frequently (compared with delavirdine that is administered three times a day).

Disadvantages:

- Use is limited to treatment-experienced patients with evidence of resistance to other agents.
- Is administered more frequently (compared with efavirenz that is administered once a day).
- Is not indicated for pediatric use (compared with efavirenz and nevirapine that are indicated for use in children as young as 3 years and 2 months, respectively).

Most important risks/adverse events:

Severe and potentially life-threatening skin reactions, including Stevens-Johnson syndrome, toxic epidermal necrolysis, erythema multiforme, and hypersensitivity reactions (treatment should be discontinued if a severe rash develops); immune reconstitution syndrome; fat redistribution; should not be included in a regimen with another NNRTI as concurrent use has not been demonstrated to be beneficial; should not be co-administered with tipranavir (Aptivus)/ritonavir, fosamprenavir (Lexiva)/ritonavir, atazanavir (Reyataz)/ritonavir, ritonavir (600 mg twice a day), or other protease inhibitors without the co-administration of low-dose ritonavir; is a substrate of the CYP3A4, CYP2C9, and CYP2C19 metabolic pathways, an inducer of CYP3A4, and an inhibitor of CYP2C9 and CYP2C19, and the concentration and activity of etravirine may be altered by the concurrent use of other agents that are substrates, inducers (e.g., carbamazepine [e.g., Tegretol], rifampin [e.g., Rifadin], St. John's wort), and inhibitors (e.g., clarithromycin [e.g., Biaxin]) of these pathways; the action of certain statins, immunosuppressants, antiarrhythmic agents, and sildenafil may be decreased by the concurrent use of etravirine, whereas the action of warfarin may be increased.

Most common adverse events:

Rash (17%), nausea (14%).

Usual dosage:

200 mg twice a day following a meal.

Product:

Tablets – 100 mg.

Comments:

Etravirine is the fourth antiretroviral agent to be classified as a NNRTI. However, it is effective in some patients with HIV-1 strains that are resistant to other NNRTIs. The effectiveness of etravirine was demonstrated in two placebo-controlled trials in patients who had already been treated with three types of antiretroviral agents (NNRTIs, nucleoside/nucleotide reverse transcriptase inhibitors [N(t)RTIs], HIV protease inhibitors). Sixty percent of those treated with etravirine plus a background antiretroviral regimen were identified as virologic responders at week 24, compared with 40% of those treated with placebo plus the background regimen.

Everolimus (Afinitor – Novartis)
Antineoplastic Agent
2009

New Drug Comparison Rating (NDCR) = 4 (significant advantages)

Indication:

Treatment of patients with advanced renal cell carcinoma after failure of treatment with sunitinib or sorafenib.

Comparable drug:

Temsirolimus (Torisel).

Advantages:

- May be effective in some patients who have not responded to sunitinib or sorafenib.
- Administered orally (whereas temsirolimus is administered intravenously).
- Less likely to cause hypersensitivity reactions.
- Lesser risk of bowel perforation, or renal failure.

Disadvantages:

- Is not a first-line treatment for advanced renal cell carcinoma.
- Available only through a restricted distribution program.

Most important risks/adverse events:

Increased risk of infection; non-infectious pneumonitis; oral ulceration (e.g., stomatitis, mucositis; management includes mouthwashes [but without alcohol or peroxide] and topical treatments); hyperlipidemias; hyperglycemia; increased creatinine; anemia; lymphopenia; use of live vaccines should be avoided; may cause harm to a fetus (Pregnancy Category D) and should not be used during pregnancy (precautions to avoid pregnancy should continue for 8 weeks following discontinuation of treatment); is a substrate of CYP3A4 (and P-glycoprotein) and action may be increased by CYP3A4 inhibitors (e.g., clarithromycin), the concurrent use of which should be avoided; action may be reduced by CYP3A4 inducers (e.g., carbamazepine) and an increase in dosage of everolimus may be necessary; is not recommended for use in patients with severe hepatic impairment.

Most common adverse events:

Oral ulceration (44%), infections (37%), asthenia (33%), fatigue (30%), cough (30%), diarrhea (30%), rash (29%), nausea (26%), anorexia (25%), peripheral edema (25%), dyspnea (24%), vomiting (20%), pyrexia (20%), anemia (92%), lymphopenia (51%), hypercholesterolemia (77%), hypertriglyceridemia (73%), hyperglycemia (57%), increased creatinine (50%).

Usual dosage:

10 mg once a day at the same time every day; in patients with moderate hepatic impairment, the recommended dosage is 5 mg once a day; this reduced dosage should also be considered in patients experiencing intolerable adverse events with the 10-mg dosage; in patients also being treated with a strong CYP3A4 inducer, an increase in dosage to 20 mg once a day (in 5-mg increments) should be considered.

Products:

Tablets – 5 mg, 10 mg; tablets should be swallowed whole, and should not be chewed or crushed.

Comments:

Everolimus inhibits the activation of mammalian target of rapamycin (mTOR), a kinase that regulates cell proliferation, cell growth, and cell survival. Its properties are most similar to those of temsirolimus, an agent that is also indicated for the treatment of advanced renal cell carcinoma and which is converted to an active metabolite, sirolimus (Rapamune), that was initially marketed for prophylaxis of organ rejection in patients receiving transplants. Although everolimus is the drug component of a drug-eluting stent, that product is considered a device and its approval for renal cell carcinoma is its first approval for use as a drug. Its effectiveness was demonstrated in studies in patients whose disease had worsened despite previous treatment with sunitinib, sorafenib, or both, sequentially. The median progression-free survival was 4.9 months in the group of patients treated with everolimus plus best supportive care compared with 1.9 months in patients receiving placebo plus best supportive care.

Many patients experience oral ulceration, for which topical treatments are recommended; however, alcohol- or peroxide-containing mouthwashes should be avoided because they may exacerbate the condition. Because everolimus has immunosuppressant properties, many patients experience infection. Patients should be advised to promptly report fever, chills, or other signs of infection.

Exenatide (Byetta – Amylin; Lilly)
Antidiabetic Agent
2005

New Drug Comparison Rating (NDCR) = 4 (significant advantages)

Indication:

Administered subcutaneously as adjunctive therapy to improve glycemic control in patients with type 2 diabetes mellitus who are taking metformin, a sulfonylurea, or a combination of metformin and a sulfonylurea but have not achieved adequate glycemic control; (subsequently revised to "as an adjunct to diet and exercise to improve glycemic control in adults with type 2 diabetes mellitus").

Comparable drugs:

Insulin (subsequent to the marketing of exenatide, sitagliptin [Januvia] and saxagliptin [Onglyza] have been marketed for the treatment of diabetes).

Advantages:

- Unique mechanism of action (mimics the action of incretins).
- May improve glycemic control in patients for whom metformin and/or a sulfonylurea have not provided adequate control (additional indications have subsequently been approved).
- Use may result in weight loss.

Disadvantages:

- Not indicated in patients with type 1 diabetes mellitus.
- Causes nausea in many patients.
- May reduce the absorption and activity of certain orally administered drugs.

Most important risks/adverse events:

Acute pancreatitis (reported in postmarketing experience); hypoglycemia (when used with a sulfonylurea and a reduction in dosage of the sulfonylurea should be considered); should not be used in patients with severe renal impairment; slows gastric emptying and may reduce the extent and rate of absorption of orally administered drugs (medications such as antibiotics and oral contraceptives that depend on threshold concentrations for effectiveness should be administered at least 1 hour before exenatide); not recommended for use in patients with severe gastrointestinal disease, including gastroparesis.

Most common adverse events:

Nausea (44%, most often when therapy is initiated), vomiting (13%), diarrhea (13%), jittery feeling (9%), dizziness (9%), headache (9%), dyspepsia (6%).

Usual dosage:

5 mcg twice a day before the morning and evening meals; after 1 month of therapy, the dosage may be increased to 10 mcg twice a day based on the clinical response.

Products:

Cartridges assembled in a pen-injector (pen) – 5 mcg, 10 mcg (should be stored in a refrigerator).

Comments:

Incretins are naturally occurring hormones that increase insulin secretion in the presence of elevated glucose concentrations (e.g., following meals). Exenatide is a synthetic form of a protein found in the saliva of the Gila monster. It mimics the action of incretins such as glucagon-like peptide-1 (GLP-1) by binding with and activating GLP-1 receptors. In addition to increasing insulin synthesis and secretion in the presence of elevated glucose concentrations, exenatide may also improve glycemic control by restoring the "first-phase" insulin response, reducing serum glucagon concentrations during periods of hyperglycemia, slowing gastric emptying, and reducing food intake. In the clinical studies, between 30% and 40% of patients treated with an exenatide regimen achieved a hemoglobin A1C of 7% or less, compared with approximately 10% of patients receiving placebo plus their previous regimen.

Unlike some antidiabetic agents (e.g., sulfonylureas, thiazolidinediones) that are often associated with weight gain, many patients treated with the higher dosage of exenatide (10 mcg twice a day) experienced a reduction in body weight. Because it may slow gastric emptying, exenatide should be used with caution in patients taking oral medications that require rapid gastrointestinal absorption (e.g., antibiotics) for optimal effectiveness.

Febuxostat (Uloric – Takeda)
Agent for Gout
2009

New Drug Comparison Rating (NDCR) = 3 (no or minor advantages/disadvantages)

Indication:
Chronic management of hyperuricemia in patients with gout.

Comparable drug:
Allopurinol (e.g., Zyloprim).

Advantages:
- Has not been reported to cause dermatologic/hypersensitivity reactions with serious complications.
- Dosage titration is less complex.
- Is administered once a day throughout the dosage range (compared with allopurinol for which dosages above 300 mg daily should be administered in divided doses).
- Dosage reduction is not necessary in patients with mild or moderate renal impairment.

Disadvantages:
- Labeled indications are more limited (allopurinol is also indicated for the management of patients with leukemia, lymphoma, and malignancies who are receiving cancer therapy which causes increased uric acid concentrations, and for the management of patients with recurrent calcium oxalate calculi).
- Is contraindicated in patients who are being treated with xanthine oxidase substrates (azathioprine [e.g., Imuran], mercaptopurine [e.g., Purinethol], theophylline); (labeling for allopurinol includes a warning about these interactions and recommendations for dosage reductions to decrease the risk of concurrent use).
- May be more likely to cause cardiovascular thromboembolic events.
- Not indicated in patients less than 18 years of age.

Most important risks/adverse events:
Contraindicated in patients being treated with azathioprine, mercaptopurine, or theophylline (the metabolism of these xanthine oxidase substrates is inhibited, resulting in increased concentrations and a risk of serious toxicity); increased gout flares; cardiovascular thromboembolic events; liver function test abnormalities (transaminase [ALT and AST] elevations; should be monitored at 2 months and 4 months, and periodically thereafter).

Most common adverse events:
Nausea (1%), arthralgia (1%), rash (1%), transaminase elevations (6%).

Usual dosage:

Initially, 40 mg once a day; in patients who do not achieve a serum uric acid concentration less than 6 mg/dL after 2 weeks with the initial dosage, the dosage should be increased to 80 mg once a day.

Products:

Tablets – 40 mg, 80 mg.

Comments:

Febuxostat is the first new treatment option for patients with chronic gout in more than 40 years. Like allopurinol, it is classified as a xanthine oxidase inhibitor. Xanthine oxidase is responsible for the breakdown of the purine base, hypoxanthine, to xanthine, and then to uric acid. Hyperuricemia is a precursor to gout. By inhibiting xanthine oxidase, febuxostat and allopurinol reduce uric acid production and lower elevated serum concentrations of uric acid. Neither febuxostat nor allopurinol is recommended for the treatment of asymptomatic hyperuricemia.

In the largest clinical study, febuxostat in a dosage of 80 mg once a day was more effective than allopurinol in a dosage of 300 mg once a day (or 200 mg once a day in patients with moderate renal impairment) in lowering serum uric acid concentrations to less than 6 mg/dL at the final visit (67% vs. 42% of patients, respectively). However, the results with febuxostat in a dosage of 40 mg once a day (45% of patients) were similar to those with allopurinol. It cannot be concluded that the new agent is more effective than allopurinol because the 300 mg/day dosage of the latter agent that was used in the clinical studies is considerably less than the maximum dosage (800 mg/day).

Following initiation of febuxostat or allopurinol treatment, gout flares may be experienced because of the mobilization of urate from tissue deposits. When initiating treatment, flare prophylaxis with a nonsteroidal anti-inflammatory drug (e.g., naproxen, 250 mg twice a day) or colchicine (0.6 mg once or twice a day) may be beneficial for up to 6 months.

Fesoterodine fumarate (Toviaz – Pfizer)
Agent for Overactive Bladder
2009

New Drug Comparison Rating (NDCR) = 3 (no or minor advantages/disadvantages)

Indication:
Treatment of overactive bladder with symptoms of urge urinary incontinence, urgency, and frequency.

Comparable drug:
Tolterodine extended-release (Detrol LA).

Advantages:
- Use in an 8 mg once-a-day dosage has been reported to be more effective than tolterodine extended-release in a 4 mg once-a-day dosage.
- May be less likely to prolong the QT interval of the electrocardiogram.

Disadvantages:
- Use in an 8 mg once-a-day dosage has been reported to cause a higher incidence of adverse events (e.g., dry mouth) than tolterodine extended release in a 4 mg once-a-day dosage.
- Not recommended for use in patients with severe hepatic impairment (tolterodine may be used in a lower dosage).

Most important risks/adverse events:
Contraindicated in patients with urinary retention, gastric retention, or uncontrolled narrow-angle glaucoma; not recommended for use in patients with severe hepatic impairment; must be used with caution in patients with bladder outlet obstruction, decreased gastrointestinal motility (e.g., those with severe constipation), myasthenia gravis, or controlled narrow-angle glaucoma; action may be increased in patients taking a potent CYP3A4 inhibitor (e.g., clarithromycin [e.g., Biaxin]) concurrently, and in patients with severe renal impairment.

Most common adverse events (and the incidences in patients receiving 8 mg once a day and 4 mg once a day, respectively):
Dry mouth (35%; 19%), constipation (6%; 4%), dry eyes (4%; 1%), dyspepsia (2%; 2%).

Usual dosage:

4 mg once a day, initially; may be increased to 8 mg once a day based on individual response and tolerability; daily dosage should not exceed 4 mg in patients with severe renal impairment or who are taking a potent CYP3A4 inhibitor concurrently.

Products:

Extended-release tablets – 4 mg, 8 mg; tablets must not be chewed, divided, or crushed.

Comments:

Fesoterodine is the sixth muscarinic receptor antagonist to be approved for the treatment of overactive bladder, joining tolterodine (e.g., Detrol LA), oxybutynin (e.g., Ditropan XL), trospium (e.g., Sanctura XR), darifenacin (Enablex), and solifenacin (Vesicare). It is most closely related to tolterodine and both drugs are converted to the same active metabolite, 5-hydroxymethyl tolterodine. Following administration, fesoterodine is rapidly and extensively hydrolyzed to this active metabolite that is responsible for the antimuscarinic activity. Its effectiveness was demonstrated in two placebo-controlled studies, and the improvement of symptoms was greater with the use of a dosage of 8 mg once a day than with the dosage of 4 mg once a day. In a study in which fesoterodine was compared with tolterodine extended-release, fesoterodine has been reported to be significantly better than tolterodine in improving a number of endpoints; however, the dosage of fesoterodine was 8 mg once a day and the dosage of tolterodine was 4 mg once a day. Although the amounts of the parent compounds and the active metabolite cannot be exactly quantified, there is considerably more active drug in an 8 mg dose of fesoterodine than in a 4 mg dose of tolterodine. This is also reflected in the higher incidence of adverse events reported with fesoterodine in this study (e.g., a 34% incidence of dry mouth with the 8 mg dose of fesoterodine compared with a 17% incidence with the 4 mg dose of tolterodine).

The most commonly experienced adverse events with both fesoterodine and tolterodine are related to their anticholinergic activity. The labeling for tolterodine, but not that for fesoterodine, includes a precaution regarding prolongation of the QT interval of the electrocardiogram.

Galsulfase (Naglazyme – BioMarin)
Agent for Mucopolysaccharidosis VI
2005

New Drug Comparison Rating (NDCR) = 5 (important advance)

Indication:
Administered via intravenous infusion for the treatment of patients with mucopolysaccharidosis VI (MPS-VI, Maroteaux-Lamy syndrome).

Comparable drugs:
None.

Advantages:
• First drug approved for mucopolysaccharidosis VI.

Disadvantages/Limitations:
• Must be administered parenterally.
• Frequency of infusion reactions.
• Available only through a restricted distribution program.

Most important risks/adverse events:
Infusion reactions (e.g., fever, rigors, headache, hypotension, angioneurotic edema).

Most common adverse events:
Abdominal pain (53%), ear pain (42%), pain (25%), conjunctivitis (21%).

Usual dosage:
1 mg/kg via intravenous infusion once a week.

Product:
Vials – 5 mg (should be stored in a refrigerator).

Comments:
Mucopolysaccharidosis VI is a rare, often fatal genetic disease characterized by the absence or marked reduction in the lysosomal hydrolase, N-acetylgalactosamine 4-sulfatase. Galsulfase is a form of this human enzyme that is produced by recombinant DNA technology, and is used as enzyme replacement therapy. It is the first drug to be approved for the treatment of mucopolysaccharidosis VI.

Golimumab (Simponi – Centocor Ortho Biotech)
Antiarthritic Agent
2009

New Drug Comparison Rating (NDCR) = 2 (significant disadvantages)

Indications:

Administered subcutaneously in adult patients for the treatment of moderately to severely active rheumatoid arthritis (in combination with methotrexate), active psoriatic arthritis (alone or in combination with methotrexate), and active ankylosing spondylitis.

Comparable drugs:

Other tumor necrosis factor (TNF) blockers: etanercept (Enbrel), adalimumab (Humira), certolizumab (Cimzia), infliximab (Remicade).

Advantages:

- Less frequent administration – once a month (compared with etanercept that is administered every week, adalimumab that is administered every two weeks, and certolizumab that is used, at least initially, every two weeks for the treatment of rheumatoid arthritis).
- Is administered subcutaneously (compared with infliximab that is administered intravenously).

Disadvantages:

- Indication for rheumatoid arthritis is more limited (indication is for use in combination with methotrexate [compared with etanercept, adalimumab, and certolizumab]; indication does not include inducing major clinical response, inhibiting progression of structural damage, and/or improving physical function [compared with etanercept, adalimumab, and infliximab]).
- Indication for psoriatic arthritis is more limited (indication does not include inhibiting the progression of structural damage or improving physical function [compared with etanercept, adalimumab, and infliximab]).
- Has not been directly compared with other agents in clinical studies.
- Fewer labeled indications (compared with etanercept that is also indicated for juvenile idiopathic arthritis and plaque psoriasis, adalimumab that is also indicated for juvenile idiopathic arthritis, plaque psoriasis, and Crohn's disease, and infliximab that is also indicated for plaque psoriasis, Crohn's disease, and ulcerative colitis).
- Is not indicated for use in patients less than 18 years of age (compared with etanercept, adalimumab, and infliximab that are used for certain indications in children).

Most important risks/adverse events:

Serious infections (boxed warning; e.g., tuberculosis [TB], invasive fungal infections, and other opportunistic infections [patients should be evaluated for TB risk factors and be tested for latent TB infection; treatment should not be initiated in patients with active infections, including clinically important localized infections; treatment should be discontinued if a patient develops a serious infection; concurrent use with abatacept (Orencia) or anakinra (Kineret) is not recommended because of the increased risk of serious infection]); malignancies (e.g., lymphomas); exacerbation or new onset of congestive heart failure; exacerbation or new onset of demyelinating disease (e.g., multiple sclerosis); hepatitis B virus reactivation; hematologic reactions; live vaccines should not be used concurrently.

Most common adverse events:

Upper respiratory tract infection (7%), nasopharyngitis (6%), injection site erythema (3%); hypertension (3%).

Usual dosage:

50 mg once a month subcutaneously.

Products:

Prefilled syringe and prefilled SmartJect autoinjector – 50 mg/0.5 mL (should be refrigerated).

Comments:

Golimumab is a humanized monoclonal antibody that prevents the binding of tumor necrosis factor (TNF) alpha to its receptors, thereby inhibiting its activity. It is the fifth TNF blocker to be marketed for the treatment of rheumatoid arthritis. As with infliximab, golimumab's indication for rheumatoid arthritis is in combination with methotrexate, whereas this limitation does not apply with the use of the other TNF blockers. In addition, the indications for golimumab for rheumatoid arthritis and psoriatic arthritis are more limited than those for etanercept, adalimumab, and infliximab, and the new drug also has fewer labeled indications than etanercept, adalimumab, and infliximab.

Ibandronate sodium (Boniva — Roche; GlaxoSmithKline)
Agent for Osteoporosis
2005

New Drug Comparison Rating (NDCR) = 4 (significant advantages)

Indication:
Treatment and prevention of osteoporosis in postmenopausal women.

Comparable drugs:
Alendronate (Fosamax), risedronate (Actonel); (another comparable drug, zoledronic acid [Reclast] has been subsequently marketed).

Advantages (pertaining to the oral formulations initially marketed):
- May be administered in a once-a-month dosage regimen that is more convenient for some patients.
- Less frequent (once-a-month) administration reduces the number of times at which a patient is at risk of upper gastrointestinal adverse events associated with administration of the drug.

Disadvantages (pertaining to the oral formulations initially marketed):
- Has fewer labeled indications (other agents are also indicated for the treatment of glucocorticoid-induced osteoporosis and Paget disease of bone, and alendronate is also indicated for increasing bone mass in men with osteoporosis).
- A longer time period (60 minutes compared with 30 minutes with the other agents) should elapse between the administration of the drug and consuming food or beverages or lying down.

Most important risks/adverse events:
Contraindicated in patients with uncorrected hypocalcemia; upper gastrointestinal effects (e.g., dysphagia, esophagitis, esophageal or gastric ulcer); musculoskeletal pain; osteonecrosis of the jaw.

Most common adverse events:
Back pain (14%), dyspepsia (12%), bronchitis (10%), abdominal pain (8%), pain in extremity (8%), diarrhea (7%), headache (7%), arthralgia (6%), myalgia (6%).

Usual dosage:
2.5 mg once a day or 150 mg once a month on the same date each month; should be administered with plain water (not mineral water) at least 60 minutes before the first food or drink of the day and before taking any oral medications or other products

containing multivalent cations (e.g., antacids, calcium supplements, milk); (Subsequent to the marketing of the tablet formulations of ibandronate, a parenteral formulation of ibandronate was approved for which the recommended dosage is 3 mg every 3 months administered intravenously over 15 to 30 seconds.)

Products:

Tablets – 2.5 mg, 150 mg; prefilled syringe (for intravenous administration) – 3 mg.

Comments:

Ibandronate is the third bisphosphonate derivative to be marketed for the treatment and prevention of osteoporosis in postmenopausal women, joining alendronate and risedronate. Another bisphosphonate, zoledronic acid, was initially marketed (Zometa) for the treatment of hypercalcemia of malignancy; in 2007 it was approved/marketed (Reclast) for the treatment of postmenopausal osteoporosis as a once-a-year intravenous infusion. The bisphosphonates inhibit osteoclast activity, reduce bone resorption and turnover, increase bone mineral density, and reduce the incidence of fractures.

The primary concern with the oral use of the bisphosphonates is the risk of upper gastrointestinal (GI) adverse events (e.g., esophageal ulceration). To reduce this risk, the transit of ibandronate through the esophagus to the stomach should be facilitated by having patients swallow the tablet whole with a full glass (6 to 8 ounces) of water while standing or sitting in an upright position. They should not lie down for at least 60 minutes following administration of the drug. There have been rare reports of osteonecrosis of the jaw (ONJ) associated with the use of the bisphosphonates, primarily with the use of high doses administered intravenously in patients with cancer; however, some of these experiences have been associated with oral use of these agents.

The oral bioavailability of the bisphosphonates is very low (approximately 0.6% for ibandronate), and may be reduced by food, beverages, and medications. Ibandronate should be administered with plain water at least 60 minutes before the first food or drink of the day and before taking any products that contain multivalent cations.

Idursulfase (Elaprase — Shire)
Agent for Hunter Syndrome
2006

New Drug Comparison Rating (NDCR) = 5 (important advance)

Indication:

Administered via intravenous infusion for the treatment of Hunter syndrome.

Comparable drugs:

None.

Advantages:

- First drug demonstrated to be effective for the treatment of Hunter syndrome (mucopolysaccharidosis type II).

Disadvantages/Limitations:

- Risk of hypersensitivity reactions.
- Must be administered intravenously.

Most important risks/adverse events:

Hypersensitivity reactions (boxed warning; hypoxic episodes, hypotension, angioedema, seizures); for patients who experience infusion reactions, subsequent infusions may be managed by use of an antihistamine and/or corticosteroid prior to or during infusions, a slower rate of infusion, and/or early discontinuation of an infusion if serious symptoms develop.

Most common adverse events:

Fever (63%), headache (59%), arthralgia (31%), limb pain (28%), pruritus (28%), hypertension (25%).

Usual dosage:

Administered by intravenous infusion over 1 to 3 hours; 0.5 mg/kg once a week.

Product:

Vials – 6 mg (should be stored in a refrigerator); must be diluted with 100 mL of 0.9% Sodium Chloride Injection; initial infusion rate should be 8 mL/hour for the first 15 minutes; if the infusion is well tolerated, the rate may be increased by 8 mL/hour increments at 15-minute intervals to administer the full volume within the desired period of time; infusion rate must not exceed 100 mL/hour.

Comments:

Hunter syndrome, also known as mucopolysaccharidosis type II or MPS II, is a rare inherited disease caused by a deficiency of the lysosomal enzyme iduronate-2-sulfatase. This enzyme cleaves terminal sulfate moieties from the glycosaminoglycans (GAGs) dermatan sulfate and heparan sulfate. In patients with a deficiency of this enzyme, GAGs progressively accumulate in the lysosomes of a variety of cells, resulting in cellular engorgement, organomegaly, tissue destruction, and organ dysfunction. Hunter syndrome is diagnosed in approximately 1 of every 100,000 births. It usually becomes apparent when children are between 1 and 3 years of age and is characterized by symptoms such as growth delay, joint stiffness, and coarsening of facial features. As the disease worsens, complications such as enlargement of the liver and spleen, respiratory and cardiac problems, and neurological deficits occur. More severe forms of the disease often result in death by age 15.

Idursulfase is a purified form of human iduronate-2-sulfatase that is produced by recombinant DNA technology. It replaces the deficient enzyme and hydrolyzes the 2-sulfate esters of terminal iduronate sulfate residues from dermatan sulfate and heparan sulfate in the lysosomes of various cell types. It is the first drug to be approved for the treatment of Hunter syndrome. Idursulfase was evaluated in a 53-week placebo-controlled trial, and patients receiving the drug on a weekly basis experienced a 35-meter greater mean increase in the distance walked in 6 minutes compared with placebo. In addition to improving walking capacity, treatment resulted in a marked reduction in mean urinary GAG concentrations, as well as a sustained reduction in both liver and spleen volumes.

A potential for hypersensitivity reactions is the most important concern with the use of idursulfase. In clinical studies, 15% of patients experienced infusion reactions that involved adverse events in at least two of the following systems: cutaneous, respiratory, and cardiovascular.

Iloperidone (Fanapt – Novartis)
Antipsychotic Agent
2009

New Drug Comparison Rating (NDCR) = 1 (important disadvantages)

Indication:
Acute treatment of adults with schizophrenia; association of the drug with prolongation of the QT interval will often lead to the conclusion that other drugs should be tried first; risk of orthostatic hypotension and syncope necessitates slow titration of dosage that delays onset of antipsychotic activity.

Comparable drugs:
Risperidone (e.g., Risperdal).

Advantages:
- Less likely to cause extrapyramidal symptoms.
- Dosage adjustment is not necessary in patients with renal impairment (whereas a lower dosage of risperidone should be used in patients with severe renal impairment).

Disadvantages:
- May be less effective, particularly during the first two weeks of treatment, corresponding to and immediately following the dosage titration period.
- Not considered a first-line treatment.
- Labeled indications are more limited (risperidone is also indicated for the maintenance treatment of schizophrenia, for the treatment of bipolar disorder, and for the treatment of irritability associated with autistic disorder).
- Greater risk of QT interval prolongation (should be avoided in patients with risk factors for this response).
- Greater risk of orthostatic hypotension, necessitating slow titration of dosage that results in a delayed onset of action.
- Not recommended in patients with hepatic impairment.
- Administered twice a day (whereas risperidone may be administered once a day).
- Effectiveness and safety have not been established in pediatric patients (whereas risperidone has indications for use in children and adolescents).
- Fewer formulation options (risperidone is also available in an oral solution, orally disintegrating tablets, and an extended-release parenteral formulation).

Most important risks/adverse events:
Increased mortality in elderly patients with dementia-related psychosis (boxed warning; is not approved for the treatment of dementia-related psychosis); cerebrovascular adverse events; QT interval prolongation (should not be used in patients at risk including those who are taking other medications that are known to cause QT prolongation [e.g., certain antiarrhythmic agents, moxifloxacin (Avelox)]); orthostatic hypotension and syncope (dosage must be slowly titrated); priapism; neuroleptic malignant syndrome; tardive dyskinesia; hyperglycemia and diabetes mellitus; leukopenia, neutropenia, and

agranulocytosis; hyperprolactinemia; disruption of body temperature regulation; dysphagia; seizures; potential for cognitive and motor impairment (patients should be cautioned about engaging in activities requiring mental alertness); suicide (risk is inherent in psychiatric illness); use is not recommended in patients with hepatic impairment; is a substrate for CYP3A4 and CYP2D6 and action may be increased by the concurrent use of other medications that inhibit these metabolic pathways; may increase the action of central nervous system depressants and antihypertensive medications.

Most common adverse events (at the incidence reported with a dosage of 20-24 mg/day):

Dizziness (20%), somnolence (15%), tachycardia (12%), dry mouth (10%), weight gain (9%), nasal congestion (8%), fatigue (6%), orthostatic hypotension (5%).

Usual dosage:

To reduce the risk of orthostatic hypotension the dosage must be titrated slowly; the recommended initial dosage is 1 mg twice a day with daily adjustments made to 2 mg twice daily, 4 mg twice daily, 6 mg twice daily, 8 mg twice daily, 10 mg twice daily, and 12 mg twice daily on days 2, 3, 4, 5, 6, and 7, respectively; the maximum recommended dosage is 12 mg twice a day; when used concomitantly with a CYP3A4 inhibitor (e.g., clarithromycin) or CYP2D6 inhibitor (e.g., paroxetine), the dosage of iloperidone should be reduced by one-half.

Products:

Tablets – 1 mg, 2 mg, 4 mg, 6 mg, 8 mg, 10 mg, 12 mg.

Comments:

Iloperidone is an atypical antipsychotic agent that is classified as a benzisoxazole derivative. Its properties are most similar to those of risperidone, paliperidone (Invega; the active metabolite of risperidone), and ziprasidone (Geodon). Other atypical antipsychotic agents include aripiprazole (Abilify), olanzapine (Zyprexa), quetiapine (Seroquel), asenapine (Saphris), and clozapine (e.g., Clozaril). The efficacy of these agents is thought to be mediated through a combination of antagonist activity at dopamine type 2 (D2) receptors and serotonin type 2 (5-HT2) receptors. In a 6-week study in which patients received iloperidone, risperidone, or placebo, the new drug was determined to be superior to placebo but less effective than risperidone, at least during the first two weeks of the study. It has been suggested that this difference in efficacy is attributable to the slow titration of dosage with iloperidone, compared with the more rapid titration that is possible with risperidone. Although the efficacy of maintenance dosages of the two agents is likely to be similar, the delay in attaining the full clinical benefit of iloperidone is an important disadvantage, particularly because it is used for the acute treatment of schizophrenia. The delayed onset of action, as well as the potential for QT interval prolongation, warrant consideration of other antipsychotic agents before using iloperidone.

When used in a dosage of 12 mg twice a day, iloperidone was associated with QTc prolongation of 9 msec although no severe cardiac arrhythmias were observed in the clinical studies. The use of the drug should be avoided in patients treated with other medications know to prolong the QT interval or who have other risk factors for QT prolongation. In patients treated with iloperidone in a dosage of 20-24 mg/day, 18% experienced at least a 7% increase in body weight, compared with 4% of those receiving placebo.

Iloprost (Ventavis – Actelion)
Agent for Pulmonary Arterial Hypertension
2005

New Drug Comparison Rating (NDCR) = 4 (significant advantages)

Indication:

Administered via inhalation for the treatment of pulmonary arterial hypertension (WHO group I) in patients with NYHA class III or IV symptoms.

Comparable drugs:

Bosentan (Tracleer), epoprostenol (Flolan), sildenafil (Revatio), treprostinil (Remodulin); (another comparable drug, ambrisentan [Letairis] was marketed in 2007).

Advantages:

- Unique route of administration (inhalation).
- More convenient to administer (compared with epoprostenol and treprostinil).
- Less likely to interact with other drugs (compared with bosentan and sildenafil).

Disadvantages:

- Less convenient to administer (compared with bosentan and sildenafil, which are administered orally).
- Available only through a restricted distribution program.

Most important risks/adverse events:

Hypotension (particularly in patients who are also being treated with other medications that lower blood pressure); pulmonary edema (treatment should be immediately discontinued); bronchospasm; increased risk of bleeding in patients on anticoagulant therapy.

Most common adverse events:

Flushing (18%), increased cough (13%), headache (10%), trismus (9%), insomnia (6%), hypotension (5%)—incidences reported represent the differences between the drug and placebo groups.

Usual dosage:

2.5 mcg (as delivered at the mouthpiece) administered via inhalation 6 to 9 times a day during waking hours, but not more than once every 2 hours; if this dose is well tolerated, the dose should be increased to 5 mcg 6 to 9 times a day; has been evaluated using two pulmonary drug delivery devices, the I-neb AAD (Adaptive Aerosol Delivery) System and the Prodose AAD System.

Products:

Ampules – 10 mcg, 20 mcg (one ampule is used for each inhalation treatment).

Comments:

Iloprost is a synthetic analogue of prostacyclin PGI2 that is administered by inhalation. Like epoprostenol and treprostinil, it dilates systemic and pulmonary arterial vascular beds. In controlled studies, it improved a composite endpoint consisting of exercise tolerance, symptoms, and lack of deterioration. However, there was not evidence of benefit in patients with pulmonary hypertension associated with chronic thromboembolic disease. The marketing of both iloprost and sildenafil (for the treatment of PAH) in 2005 and ambrisentan in 2007 increases the number of agents providing benefit in the treatment of PAH via different mechanisms of action, thereby offering a potential for attaining greater benefit with combination regimens than with any of the agents given alone.

Because of possible drug delivery device malfunction, it is recommended that patients have ready access to a back-up system.

Insulin detemir (Levemir – Novo Nordisk)
Antidiabetic Agent
2006

New Drug Comparison Rating (NDCR) = 2 (significant disadvantages)

Indication:
Once- or twice-daily subcutaneous administration for the treatment of adult and pediatric patients with type 1 diabetes mellitus or adult patients with type 2 diabetes mellitus who require basal (long-acting) insulin for the control of hyperglycemia.

Comparable drugs:
Insulin glargine (Lantus).

Advantages:
None.

Disadvantages:
- Duration of action may be shorter and twice-daily administration may be necessary for optimum glycemic control.
- Less flexibility in the time of administration when administered once a day (insulin glargine may be administered at any time during the day [at the same time every day]).

Most important risks/adverse events:
Hypoglycemia (concurrent use of other medications that may alter glucose concentrations should be closely monitored).

Most common adverse events:
Pruritus, injection site reactions, weight gain.

Usual dosage:
Administered subcutaneously and dosage should be individualized; when used once a day should be administered with the evening meal or at bedtime; when used twice a day the first dose is administered in the morning, and the second dose with the evening meal, at bedtime, or 12 hours after the morning dose.

Products:
Solution – 100 units/mL, supplied in vials, PenFill cartridges, and prefilled syringes (should be stored in a refrigerator).

Comments:

Insulin detemir is a human insulin analogue that is produced by recombinant DNA technology. It is classified as a long-acting insulin, as is insulin glargine. However, it has a shorter duration of action than insulin glargine and, in some patients, it should be administered twice a day. In the clinical study in which the two agents were directly compared, insulin detemir was administered twice a day whereas insulin glargine was administered once a day.

Insulin glulisine (Apidra – Sanofi-Aventis)
Antidiabetic Agent
2006

New Drug Comparison Rating (NDCR) = 2 (significant disadvantages)

Indication:

For subcutaneous administration for the treatment of adult patients with diabetes mellitus for the control of hyperglycemia (has been subsequently approved for use in patients 4 -17 years of age).

Comparable drugs:

Insulin aspart (NovoLog), insulin lispro (Humalog).

Advantages:

None.

Disadvantages:

- Indication is only for adult patients (indication for insulin lispro is not limited to adults); (has been subsequently approved for use in patients 4-17 years of age).
- Indication does not include concurrent use with a sulfonylurea (indication for insulin lispro includes use in combination with a sulfonylurea antidiabetic agent instead of a longer-acting insulin in patients with type 2 diabetes).
- Not available in a combination formulation with a longer-acting insulin (insulin aspart and insulin lispro are available in combination formulations that also include insulin aspart protamine and insulin lispro protamine, respectively).
- Is in Pregnancy Category C (insulin lispro is in Category B).

Most important risks/adverse events:

Hypoglycemia (concurrent use with other medications that may alter glucose concentrations should be closely monitored).

Most common adverse events:

Pruritus, injection site reactions, weight gain.

Usual dosage:

Administered subcutaneously and dosage should be individualized; doses should be administered within 15 minutes before a meal or within 20 minutes after starting a meal.

Products:

Solution – 100 units/mL, supplied in vials and cartridges (should be stored in a refrigerator); cartridges are for use only in the OptiClik insulin delivery device.

Comments:

Insulin glulisine is a human insulin analogue that is produced by recombinant DNA technology. It has a rapid onset of action and short duration of action, and its properties are most similar to those of insulin aspart and insulin lispro. Each of the three agents is administered at mealtimes. The three agents may also be administered subcutaneously by external infusion pumps.

If insulin glulisine is mixed with NPH insulin, the new agent should be drawn into the syringe first and the injection should be administered immediately after mixing. Both insulin lispro and insulin aspart are also available in combination with their protamine forms that have an intermediate duration of action, and are designated as Humalog Mix 75/25 and NovoLog Mix 70/30, respectively.

Ixabepilone (Ixempra — Bristol-Myers Squibb)
Antineoplastic Agent
2007

New Drug Comparison Rating (NDCR) = 4 (significant advantages)

Indications:

Administered via intravenous infusion, in a combination regimen with capecitabine (Xeloda), for the treatment of metastatic or locally advanced breast cancer in patients after failure of an anthracycline and a taxane; also indicated as monotherapy for the treatment of metastatic or locally advanced breast cancer in patients after failure of an anthracycline, a taxane, and capecitabine.

Comparable drugs:

Lapatinib (Tykerb).

Advantages:

- May be effective in some patients with breast cancer who do not respond, or no longer respond, to other therapies.
- Use is not limited to patients whose tumors overexpress HER2.
- Less likely to cause cardiovascular adverse events.

Disadvantages:

- Must be administered intravenously (lapatinib is administered orally).
- Greater risk of toxicity and neutropenia-related death in patients with hepatic impairment.
- More likely to cause peripheral neuropathy.
- More likely to cause hypersensitivity reactions.

Most important risks/adverse events:

Myelosuppression, primarily neutropenia (contraindicated in patients with a baseline neutrophil count less than 1500 cells/mm^3 or a platelet count less than 100,000 cells/mm^3; peripheral blood counts should be frequently monitored); increased risk of toxicity and neutropenia-related death when used in combination with capecitabine in patients with hepatic impairment (boxed warning; must not be used in patients with AST or ALT greater than 2.5 times the upper limit of normal [ULN] or bilirubin greater than 1 x ULN); peripheral neuropathy, primarily sensory; hypersensitivity reactions (patients should be premedicated prior to infusion; use is contraindicated in patients with a history of hypersensitivity to products formulated with Cremophor EL); may cause harm to a fetus and use should be avoided during pregnancy; is a substrate for CYP3A4 (concurrent use with a strong CYP3A4 inhibitor [e.g., clarithromycin (e.g., Biaxin)] should be avoided; if use cannot be avoided, the dosage of ixabepilone should be reduced); concurrent use of St. John's wort should be avoided.

Most common adverse events:

Peripheral neuropathy (62%), fatigue/asthenia (56%), myalgia/arthralgia (49%), alopecia (48%), nausea (42%), vomiting (29%), stomatitis/mucositis (29%), diarrhea (22%), musculoskeletal pain (20%); additional adverse events that were commonly reported with use in combination with capecitabine include palmar-plantar erythrodysesthesia syndrome (64%), anorexia (34%), abdominal pain (24%), nail disorder (24%), constipation (22%).

Usual dosage:

Administered via intravenous infusion over 3 hours; 40 mg/m^2 every 3 weeks; dosage for patients with a body surface area greater than 2.2 m^2 should be calculated based on 2.2 m^2; dosage should be reduced in patients who are also being treated with a strong CYP3A4 inhibitor, and should be adjusted in patients who experience significant adverse events (e.g., hematologic, neuropathy).

Products:

Vials – 15 mg, 45 mg, supplied in kits that also provide vials of diluent (should be stored in a refrigerator); diluent is a solution of polyoxyethylated castor oil (e.g., Cremophor EL) and dehydrated alcohol; constituted solution should be diluted with Lactated Ringer's Injection supplied in DEHP (di-[2-ethylhexyl]phthalate)-free bags; DEHP-free infusion containers and administration sets must be used (subsequently revised to include 0.9 % Sodium Chloride Injection and PLASMA-LYTE A injection pH 7.4 as qualified diluents).

Comments:

Ixabepilone is a semisynthetic analog of epothilone B that acts as a microtubule inhibitor. The drug binds directly to beta-tubulin subunits on microtubules, resulting in suppression of microtubule dynamics. In combination regimens ixabepilone provided a significant improvement in progression-free survival. As monotherapy, clinically significant tumor shrinkage occurred in 12% of patients.

Lacosamide (Vimpat – UCB)
Antiepileptic Drug
2009

New Drug Comparison Rating (NDCR) = 4 (significant advantages)

Indication:

Adjunctive therapy in the treatment of partial-onset seizures in patients with epilepsy aged 17 years and older; injection for intravenous use may be used when oral administration is temporarily not feasible.

Comparable drugs:

Carbamazepine (e.g., Tegretol), oxcarbazepine (Trileptal), lamotrigine (e.g., Lamictal), levetiracetam (e.g., Keppra).

Advantages:

- Has reduced seizure frequency in some patients in whom previous treatment did not provide adequate seizure control.
- Has a unique mechanism of action.
- Less likely to cause serious adverse events (compared with carbamazepine that has a boxed warning regarding serious dermatological reactions, aplastic anemia, and agranulocytosis, lamotrigine that has a boxed warning regarding serious rashes, and oxcarbazepine that may cause serious dermatological reactions and anaphylaxis/angioedema).
- Less likely to interact with other drugs (compared with carbamazepine).
- Less risk if used during pregnancy (is in Pregnancy Category C compared with carbamazepine that is in Category D).
- Available in a formulation for intravenous use when oral administration is not feasible (compared with carbamazepine, oxcarbazepine, and lamotrigine).

Disadvantages:

- Is not indicated for use as monotherapy (compared with carbamazepine, oxcarbazepine, and lamotrigine).
- Is not indicated for use in patients less than 17 years of age (levetiracetam is indicated for use in children as young as 4 years of age, lamotrigine and oxcarbazepine in children as young as 2 years of age, and there has been extensive experience with carbamazepine in pediatric patients).
- Labeled indications are more limited (compared with carbamazepine that is also indicated for generalized tonic-clonic seizures, mixed seizure patterns, bipolar disorder, and trigeminal neuralgia, lamotrigine that is also indicated for tonic-clonic seizures, Lennox-Gastaut syndrome, and bipolar disorder, and levetiracetam that is also indicated for tonic-clonic seizures and myoclonic seizures).
- Is a controlled substance (Schedule V).
- May prolong the PR interval of the electrocardiogram.
- Is administered twice a day (compared with formulations of levetiracetam [Keppra XR] and lamotrigine [Lamictal XR] that are administered once a day).

Most important risks/adverse events:

Suicidal ideation and behavior (patients should be monitored for the emergence or worsening of depression, suicidal thoughts, and/or unusual changes in mood or behavior); central nervous system (CNS) effects (e.g., dizziness, fatigue, ataxia; patients should be advised not to engage in potentially hazardous activities until they have assessed whether the drug adversely affects their mental and/or motor performance, and cautioned about the added risk if other CNS depressants, including alcoholic beverages, are used concurrently); syncope; prolongation of PR interval (caution is advised in patients with cardiac conduction problems, severe cardiac disease [e.g., myocardial ischemia, heart failure], or who are taking other drugs that prolong the PR interval [e.g., calcium channel blockers]); multiorgan hypersensitivity reactions (e.g., nephritis, hepatitis).

Most common adverse events:

Dizziness (30%), headache (14%), nausea (11%), vomiting (9%), diplopia (11%), blurred vision (9%), somnolence (8%), ataxia (7%), fatigue (7%).

Usual dosage:

50 mg twice a day initially; dosage can be increased at weekly intervals by 100 mg/day given as two divided doses up to the recommended maintenance dosage of 100 to 200 mg twice a day; a dosage of 300 mg/day should not be exceeded in patients with severe renal impairment or mild to moderate hepatic impairment; use in patients with severe hepatic impairment is not recommended; formulations for oral use and intravenous infusion (over a period of 30 to 60 minutes) may be used in the same dosage; if treatment is to be discontinued, should be withdrawn gradually over a period of at least one week.

Products:

Tablets – 50 mg, 100 mg, 150 mg, 200 mg; vials – 200 mg in 20 mL of solution; parenteral formulation may be used without dilution or may be mixed with a diluent (Sodium Chloride Injection 0.9%, Dextrose Injection 5%, Lactated Ringer's Injection).

Comments:

Partial-onset seizures are usually treated with a combination of antiepileptic drugs (AEDs), and carbamazepine, lamotrigine, levetiracetam, and oxcarbazepine are often considered to be among the first-line treatment options. However, numerous other AEDs have also been used effectively in these seizure disorders. Lacosamide is a functionalized amino acid that is thought to selectively enhance slow inactivation of voltage-gated sodium channels, resulting in stabilization of hyperexcitable neuronal membranes. In addition, it binds to collapsin response mediator protein-2, although whether this binding contributes to a reduction in seizures is not known.

The effectiveness of lacosamide was demonstrated in three 12-week, placebo-controlled studies in patients who were not adequately controlled with 1 to 3 concomitant AEDs. Of the patients treated with lacosamide (400 mg/day), 40% experienced a 50% or greater reduction in seizure frequency, compared to 23% of the patients receiving placebo with concomitant AEDs.

Like other AEDs, lacosamide may increase the risk of suicidal thoughts or behavior, and patients should be closely monitored. CNS effects are common and patients should be cautioned about the pertinent risks.

Higher doses of lacosamide have produced euphoria-type responses similar to those associated with alprazolam (e.g., Xanax). The incidence of euphoria reported as an adverse event in the clinical studies is less than 1%. However, as with pregabalin (Lyrica), lacosamide has been classified in Schedule V under the provisions of the Controlled Substances Act.

Lanreotide acetate (Somatuline Depot – Ipsen; Tercica)
Agent for Acromegaly
2007

New Drug Comparison Rating (NDCR) = 3 (no or minor advantages/disadvantages)

Indication:
Administered by deep subcutaneous injection for the long-term treatment of acromegalic patients who have had an inadequate response to surgery and/or radiotherapy, or for whom surgery and/or radiotherapy is not an option.

Comparable drugs:
Octreotide (e.g., Sandostatin LAR Depot).

Advantages:
- Formulation is in a prefilled syringe that does not require reconstitution (compared with the octreotide depot formulation that requires reconstitution).
- Is administered via deep subcutaneous injection (compared with the octreotide depot formulation that is administered intramuscularly).

Disadvantages:
- Has not been directly compared with octreotide in clinical studies.
- Fewer labeled indications (octreotide is also indicated for the treatment of severe diarrhea and flushing episodes associated with metastatic carcinoid tumors and for the treatment of the profuse watery diarrhea associated with vasoactive intestinal peptide tumors [VIPomas]).
- Less flexibility with respect to formulation options and routes of administration (a short-acting formulation of octreotide is also available that is administered subcutaneously or intravenously).

Most important risks/adverse events:
May reduce gallbladder motility and facilitate gallstone formation; hyperglycemia and hypoglycemia (blood glucose concentrations should be monitored); bradycardia (caution should be exercised when initiating treatment in patients with bradycardia); may reduce the bioavailability of cyclosporine (e.g., Neoral) and necessitate an adjustment of dosage of cyclosporine.

Most common adverse events:
Diarrhea (42%), abdominal pain (17%), cholelithiasis (17%), anemia (14%), injection-site pain/inflammation/mass (11%).

Usual dosage:

Administered via deep subcutaneous injection in the superior external quadrant of the buttock; 90 mg every 4 weeks; an initial dosage of 60 mg every 4 weeks is recommended in patients with hepatic or renal impairment; subsequent dosage adjustments should be based on growth hormone and/or insulin-like growth factor-1 (IGF-1) concentrations.

Products:

Syringes – 60 mg, 90 mg, 120 mg; (should be stored in a refrigerator).

Comments:

Acromegaly is characterized by excessive secretion of growth hormone (GH) from the pituitary gland, usually from a benign tumor in the pituitary. The increased secretion of GH results in the overproduction of insulin-like growth factor (IGF-1) and excessive growth. The goal of treatment is to reduce GH and IGF-1 concentrations to normal, and treatment options include surgical removal of the tumor, radiation therapy of the pituitary gland, and drug therapy. One of the drug therapy options has been the somatostatin analog octreotide, which acts similarly to the naturally occurring hormone somatostatin and inhibits production and secretion of GH.

Lanreotide is a synthetic octapeptide analog of somatostatin with properties that are similar to those of octreotide. Its effectiveness was demonstrated in two clinical trials involving a total of 400 patients. Although lanreotide was not compared with octreotide directly, numerous patients had been previously treated with octreotide and, after a 12-week washout period, were subsequently treated with lanreotide. The efficacy of the two agents appears generally similar, with treatment goals being attained with both agents in most patients.

Lanreotide is supplied in ready-to-use, prefilled syringes and is administered via deep subcutaneous injection, whereas the depot formulation of octreotide must be reconstituted and is administered intramuscularly.

Lapatinib (Tykerb – GlaxoSmithKline)
Antineoplastic Agent
2007

New Drug Comparison Rating (NDCR) = 4 (significant advantages)

Indication:

In combination with capecitabine (Xeloda) for the treatment of patients with advanced or metastatic breast cancer whose tumors overexpress HER2 and who have received prior therapy including an anthracycline (e.g., doxorubicin), a taxane (e.g., docetaxel), and trastuzumab.

Comparable drugs:

Trastuzumab (Herceptin).

Advantages:

- May be effective in some patients with advanced breast cancer who do not respond, or no longer respond, to other therapies.
- Cross-resistance does not appear to exist.
- Is effective following oral administration (trastuzumab is administered intravenously).
- Is less likely to cause hypersensitivity reactions.

Disadvantages:

- Is not indicated for first-line use.
- Data are not yet available to demonstrate prolongation of survival.
- Is associated with a greater risk if used during pregnancy.
- Is only available through a restricted distribution program.

Most important risks/adverse events:

Hepatotoxicity (boxed warning); decreased left ventricular ejection fraction (should be determined at baseline and during treatment); interstitial lung disease and pneumonitis; QT interval prolongation; severe diarrhea; may cause harm to a fetus and should not be used during pregnancy; is a substrate for CYP3A4 and its action may be increased by the concurrent use of a CYP3A4 inhibitor (e.g., clarithromycin [e.g., Biaxin]), and decreased by the concurrent use of a CYP3A4 inducer (e.g., rifampin [e.g., Rifadin]).

Most common adverse events:

Diarrhea (65%), palmar-plantar erythrodysesthesia (i.e., hand-foot syndrome; 53%), nausea (44%), rash (28%), vomiting (26%).

Usual dosage:

Should be administered at least one hour before or one hour after a meal, and the daily dose should not be divided; 1,250 mg (5 tablets) once a day on Days 1-21 continuously in combination with capecitabine 2,000 mg/m^2/day (administered orally in 2 doses approximately 12 hours apart) on Days 1-14 in a repeating 21-day cycle; in patients with severe hepatic impairment, a reduction in dosage to 750 mg/day should be considered; if it is necessary to use a strong CYP3A4 inhibitor concurrently, a reduction in dosage to 500 mg/day should be considered; if it is necessary to use a strong CYP3A4 inducer concurrently, the dosage may be gradually increased up to 4,500 mg/day based on tolerability.

Product:

Tablets – 250 mg.

Comments:

Lapatinib is a kinase inhibitor of the intracellular tyrosine kinase domains of both Epidermal Growth Factor Receptor (EGFR [ErbB1]) and of Human Epidermal Receptor 2 (HER2 [ErbB2]) receptors. Whereas trastuzumab is a large protein molecule that targets the part of the HER2 protein on the outside of the cell (i.e., the extracellular domain), lapatinib is a small molecule that enters the cell (i.e., the intracellular domain) and blocks the function of the HER2 protein as well as other proteins. Lapatinib has been effective in some patients who have not responded, or are no longer responding, to trastuzumab or other agents. An additive effect has been demonstrated when lapatinib is used in combination with capecitabine. In the clinical studies, a combination regimen of lapatinib and capecitabine was compared with capecitabine alone. The median time to tumor progression (or death related to breast cancer) for the combination regimen was 27 weeks compared with 19 weeks for capecitabine alone. In addition, the tumor response rate was higher with the combination regimen (24% compared with 14%).

Lenalidomide (Revlimid — Celgene)
Antineoplastic Agent
2006

New Drug Comparison Rating (NDCR) = 4 (significant advantages)

Indications:

Treatment of patients with transfusion-dependent anemia due to low- or intermediate-1-risk myelodysplastic syndromes (MDS) associated with a deletion 5q cytogenetic abnormality with or without additional cytogenetic abnormalities; (subsequently approved for use in combination with dexamethasone for the treatment of patients with multiple myeloma who have received at least one prior therapy).

Comparable drugs:

Azacitidine (Vidaza).

Note: Although lenalidomide is an analogue of thalidomide (Thalomid) and both agents are now indicated for the treatment of multiple myeloma, it was initially approved for the treatment of a specific type of MDS and its NDCR is based on a comparison with azacitidine. Decitabine (Dacogen) was approved later in 2006 for the treatment of MDS.

Advantages:

- Is highly effective in attaining transfusion independence in patients with deletion 5q MDS.
- Is administered orally (azacitidine is administered subcutaneously or intravenously).

Disadvantages:

- Indication for MDS is more limited (azacitidine is indicated for any of the MDS subtypes).
- Risk of deep venous thrombosis and pulmonary embolism.
- Available only through a restricted distribution program.

Most important risks/adverse events:

Birth defects (boxed warning — use is contraindicated during pregnancy [Pregnancy Category X] and use is restricted to patients who are registered and meet the conditions of the restricted distribution program); hematologic toxicity (boxed warning — e.g., neutropenia, thrombocytopenia; complete blood counts should be monitored weekly for the first 8 weeks of therapy and at least monthly thereafter); deep venous thrombosis and pulmonary embolism (boxed warning).

Most common adverse events:

Diarrhea (49%), pruritus (42%), rash (36%), fatigue (31%), thrombocytopenia (62%), neutropenia (59%).

Usual dosage:

MDS – 10 mg once a day with water; multiple myeloma – 25 mg once a day with water on days 1 to 21 of repeated 28-day cycles.

Products:

Capsules – 5 mg, 10 mg; subsequently also marketed in a 25 mg potency.

Comments:

Myelodysplastic syndromes (MDS) comprise a group of disorders in which the bone marrow does not function normally. Deletion 5q MDS is a subtype of the disorder that is associated with a chromosome problem in which part of chromosome 5 is missing. Patients with this MDS subtype usually experience anemia that requires transfusions. Lenalidomide is an analogue of thalidomide that has immunomodulatory, antiangiogenic, and antineoplastic properties. In studies of its use in patients with deletion 5q MDS, transfusion independence (the absence of any red blood cell transfusion during any consecutive 8 weeks during the treatment period) was attained in 67% of the patients, with 90% of these patients experiencing the benefit within 3 months of initiation of therapy. The transfusion-free period lasted an average of 44 weeks.

In mid-2006, thalidomide and then lenalidomide were approved for the treatment of patients with multiple myeloma. Both agents are indicated for use in combination with dexamethasone (e.g., Decadron). However, thalidomide is indicated for use in patients with newly diagnosed multiple myeloma, whereas lenalidomide is indicated for patients who have received at least one prior therapy.

Although data are limited, lenalidomide is considered to have the known risk of thalidomide in causing severe, life-threatening birth defects if it is used during pregnancy. To reduce this risk, prescribers, pharmacists, and patients must comply with the provisions of a restricted distribution program.

Lisdexamfetamine dimesylate (Vyvanse – Shire)
Agent for Attention Deficit/Hyperactivity Disorder
2007

New Drug Comparison Rating (NDCR) = 3 (no or minor advantages/disadvantages)

Indication:

Treatment of attention deficit/hyperactivity disorder (ADHD); indicated as part of a total treatment program for ADHD that may include other measures (e.g., psychological, educational, social); (initially approved for children 6-12 years of age and subsequently approved for use in adults).

Comparable drugs:

Dextroamphetamine (e.g., Dexedrine), amphetamine/dextroamphetamine mixed salts (e.g., Adderall, Adderall XR).

Advantages:

- Formulation may have a lesser potential for abuse.
- May be administered in water for children who have difficulty swallowing capsules (compared with dextroamphetamine).
- Has a longer duration of action that permits once-daily administration (compared with Adderall).

Disadvantages:

- Has not been directly compared in clinical studies with other amphetamine/ dextroamphetamine products.
- Is not indicated in patients younger than 6 or older than 12 years of age (compared with dextroamphetamine and Adderall that have been studied in children as young as 3 years of age, and with dextroamphetamine and Adderall XR that have been studied in patients older than 12 years); (has been subsequently approved for use in older patients).
- Labeled indications are more limited (compared with dextroamphetamine and Adderall XR that are also indicated for the treatment of narcolepsy).

Most important risks/adverse events:

Potential for dependence and misuse/abuse (boxed warning; classified in Schedule II of the Controlled Substances Act); sudden death and serious cardiovascular adverse events (boxed warning with respect to the greater risk associated with misuse/abuse); psychiatric adverse events (e.g., hearing voices, becoming suspicious for no reason, becoming manic); exacerbation of motor and phonic tics and Tourette's syndrome; long-term suppression of growth; contraindicated in patients with advanced arteriosclerosis, symptomatic cardiovascular disease, moderate to severe hypertension, hyperthyroidism, or glaucoma, in patients in an agitated state or with a history of drug abuse, or during or within 14 days following the administration of a monoamine oxidase inhibitor; action may be increased by urinary alkalinizing agents, and decreased by urinary acidifying agents; may reduce the action of antihypertensive agents.

Most common adverse events:

Decreased appetite (39%), insomnia (19%), upper abdominal pain (12%), irritability (10%), vomiting (9%), decreased weight (9%), nausea (6%), dizziness (5%), dry mouth (5%).

Usual dosage:

30 mg once a day in the morning; if needed, dosage may be increased in increments of 20 mg/day and at approximately weekly intervals to the maximum recommended dosage of 70 mg/day; afternoon doses should be avoided because of the increased likelihood of insomnia; capsules may be swallowed whole or the contents of a capsule may be dissolved in a glass of water.

Products:

Capsules – 20 mg, 30 mg, 40 mg, 50 mg, 60 mg, 70 mg.

Comments:

Lisdexamfetamine is a prodrug of dextroamphetamine in which the amino acid l-lysine is linked to dextroamphetamine. Following oral administration lisdexamfetamine is rapidly absorbed and converted to dextroamphetamine, which is responsible for its activity.

Because lisdexamfetamine itself is inactive and its conversion to dextroamphetamine occurs gradually, it has been suggested that it has a lesser potential for misuse/abuse and that abuse via inhalation or intravenous use will be limited. However, it has not been demonstrated to have a lesser abuse liability and, like the related products, it is classified in Schedule II.

Lubiprostone (Amitiza – Sucampo; Takeda)
Agent for Constipation
2006

New Drug Comparison Rating (NDCR) = 4 (significant advantages)

Indication:
Treatment of chronic idiopathic constipation in adults; (has been subsequently approved for the treatment of irritable bowel syndrome with constipation in women 18 years of age and older).

Comparable drugs:
Tegaserod (Zelnorm); (See Comments).

Advantages:
- Has a unique mechanism of action.
- Indication is not restricted to use in adults less than 65 years of age (an initial restriction with tegaserod).
- Effectiveness has been demonstrated over treatment periods of up to 12 months (compared to 12 weeks with tegaserod).
- Less likely to cause problems in patients with severe renal impairment or moderate or severe hepatic impairment (in whom tegaserod is contraindicated).
- May be less likely to cause complications associated with diarrhea.

Disadvantages:
- More likely to cause nausea.
- More likely to cause harm to a fetus.

Most important risks/adverse events:
Contraindicated in patients with a history of mechanical gastrointestinal obstruction; dyspnea; animal studies suggest a potential for causing fetal loss and women who could become pregnant should have a negative pregnancy test prior to initiating therapy and should use effective contraceptive measures.

Most common adverse events:
Nausea (31%), diarrhea (13%), headache (13%), abdominal distension (7%), abdominal pain (7%), flatulence (6%).

Usual dosage:
Chronic idiopathic constipation - 24 mcg twice a day with food and water; irritable bowel syndrome with constipation – 8 mcg twice a day with food and water.

Product:

Capsules – 8 mcg, 24 mcg.

Comments:

Chronic idiopathic constipation is a common disorder that is experienced over a period of more than 6 months, more often by women than men, and more often in those over 65 years of age. Dietary fiber and laxatives may be of benefit but these approaches are of limited value in many patients. Tegaserod is a serotonin 5-HT4 receptor partial agonist that was initially approved for the treatment of irritable bowel syndrome associated with constipation, and subsequently as the first drug to be specifically approved for the treatment of chronic idiopathic constipation in adults less than 65 years of age. However, the marketing of tegaserod was suspended in early 2007 because of concerns regarding a potentially higher risk of heart attack, stroke, and unstable angina. In July, 2007 the availability of tegaserod was resumed on a restricted basis under a treatment investigational new drug protocol for women younger than 55 who meet specific guidelines. However, in April 2008, this restricted access program was discontinued.

Lubiprostone is a chloride channel activator that acts locally to activate C1C-2, which is a normal constituent of the apical membrane of the intestinal epithelium. Its use provides a chloride-rich intestinal fluid secretion without altering sodium and potassium concentrations in the serum. By increasing intestinal fluid secretion, lubiprostone increases motility in the intestine, thereby facilitating the passage of stool and alleviating symptoms associated with constipation. It is the second drug to be approved for the treatment of chronic idiopathic constipation and its use is not restricted, as is the situation with tegaserod.

Lubiprostone has low systemic availability and its actions are primarily localized in the gastrointestinal tract. Administration of the drug with food decreases the occurrence of nausea.

Maraviroc (Selzentry – Pfizer)
Antiviral Agent
2007

New Drug Comparison Rating (NDCR) = 4 (significant advantages)

Indication:

In combination with other antiretroviral agents, for treatment-experienced adult patients infected with only CCR5-tropic HIV-1 detectable, who have evidence of viral replication and HIV-1 strains resistant to multiple antiretroviral agents (subsequently revised to delete restriction to treatment-experienced patients).

Comparable drug:

Enfuvirtide (Fuzeon).

Advantages:

- Has a unique mechanism of action (inhibits entry of CCR5-tropic HIV-1 into cells).
- Is effective in some patients who have become resistant to previous regimens.
- Is administered orally (enfuvirtide is administered subcutaneously).

Disadvantages:

- Does not inhibit the entry of CXCR4-tropic and dual tropic HIV-1 into cells.
- Greater risk of causing hepatic adverse events.
- Interacts with more medications.

Most important risks/adverse events:

Hepatotoxicity (boxed warning), which may be preceded by evidence of a systemic allergic reaction (e.g., pruritic rash); caution should be exercised in patients with pre-existing liver dysfunction or who are co-infected with viral hepatitis B or C; immune reconstitution syndrome; increased risk of infection; use with caution in patients at increased risk for cardiovascular events; risk of adverse events is increased in patients with impaired renal function; is a substrate for CYP3A and action may be increased by the concurrent use of CYP3A inhibitors (e.g., HIV protease inhibitors [except tipranavir/ritonavir]), delavirdine [Rescriptor], clarithromycin [e.g., Biaxin]), and decreased by the concurrent use of CYP3A inducers (e.g., efavirenz [Sustiva], rifampin [e.g., Rifadin]); should not be used concurrently with St. John's wort.

Most common adverse events:

Upper respiratory tract infection (20%), cough (13%), pyrexia (12%), rash (10%), musculoskeletal symptoms (9%), abdominal pain (8%), dizziness (8%).

Usual dosage:

300 mg twice a day; a dosage of 150 mg twice a day is recommended in patients also being treated with a CYP3A inhibitor (with or without a CYP3A inducer); a dosage of 600 mg twice a day is recommended in patients also being treated with a CYP3A inducer (without a strong CYP3A inhibitor).

Products:

Tablets – 150 mg, 300 mg.

Comments:

With only one exception (enfuvirtide [Fuzeon]), the previously marketed antiretroviral agents inhibit HIV replication within white cells. Enfuvirtide interferes with the entry of HIV into cells by inhibiting fusion of viral and cellular membranes, and is designated as a fusion inhibitor. CCR5 is a chemokine receptor protein that is present on the surface of some immune cells and is the primary route by which HIV-1 enters uninfected cells. Maraviroc has a unique mechanism of action and is classified as a CCR5 co-receptor antagonist. It selectively binds to CCR5 that is necessary for CCR5-tropic HIV-1 to enter cells, thereby inhibiting the entry of virus into cells. Approximately 60% of patients who have already received antiretroviral medications have circulating CCR5-tropic HIV-1. Maraviroc does not appear to inhibit cell entry via the other HIV-1 co-receptor CXCR4 or dual-entry-tropic HIV-1. The identification of patients for whom maraviroc treatment is appropriate should be guided by tropism testing (i.e., Trofile HIV coreceptor tropism assay).

The effectiveness of maraviroc in reducing HIV-1 RNA concentrations was demonstrated in two controlled studies in patients who had already been treated with three classes of antiretroviral agents who had evidence of HIV-1 replication despite ongoing treatment. Patients received either maraviroc or placebo in addition to optimized background therapy consisting of three to six antiretroviral agents. The action of maraviroc is additive/synergistic with enfuvirtide.

Mecasermin (Increlex – Tercica)
Agent for Growth Failure
2006

New Drug Comparison Rating (NDCR) = 5 (important advance)

Indication:
Administered subcutaneously for the long-term treatment of growth failure in children with severe primary IGF-1 deficiency (Primary IGFD) or with growth hormone gene deletion who have developed neutralizing antibodies to growth hormone.

Comparable drugs:
None.

Advantages:
- First drug to be approved for the treatment of growth failure in children with severe primary insulin-like growth factor-1 (IGF-1) deficiency or with growth hormone gene deletion who have developed neutralizing antibodies to growth hormone.

Disadvantages/Limitations:
- Frequency of hypoglycemia.

Most important risks/adverse events:
Contraindicated in patients with closed epiphyses, and in the presence of active or suspected neoplasia; hypoglycemia (should be administered shortly before or after [20 minutes on either side of] a meal or snack); local or systemic allergic reactions; lymphoid tissue (e.g., tonsillar) hypertrophy; intracranial hypertension; slipped capital femoral epiphysis; worsening of scoliosis.

Most common adverse events:
Hypoglycemia (42%), tonsillar hypertrophy (15%), and the following adverse events in at least 5% of patients—snoring, otitis media, ear pain, fluid in middle ear, headache, dizziness, convulsions, vomiting, cardiac murmur, arthralgia, pain in extremity, bruising, lipohypertrophy.

Usual dosage:
Administered subcutaneously within 20 minutes before or after a meal or snack (should not be administered when the meal or snack is omitted); recommended initial dosage is 0.04 to 0.08 mg/kg twice a day; if this dosage is well tolerated for at least 1 week, the dosage may be increased by 0.04 mg/kg/dose to the maximum dosage of 0.12 mg/kg twice a day; subcutaneous injection sites should be rotated to a different site with each injection.

117

Product:

Vials – 10 mg/mL (40 mg/vial); (should be stored in a refrigerator).

Comments:

Some children of short stature have normal or elevated concentrations of growth hormone and would not be expected to benefit from treatment with growth hormone. Insulin-like growth factor-1 (IGF-1) is the primary mediator of statural growth, and a deficiency of this hormone is responsible for some children failing to grow at the expected rate. Severe primary deficiencies of IGF may result from mutations in the growth hormone receptor, post-growth hormone receptor signaling pathway, and IGF-1 gene defects. Mecasermin is human IGF-1 produced by recombinant DNA technology and is the first drug to be approved for the treatment of growth failure in children with severe primary IGF-1 deficiency. In the clinical studies in which it was compared with pretreatment growth patterns, children treated with mecasermin gained, on average, an additional inch per year for each year of therapy. The drug has not been studied in children under 2 years of age or in adults.

Because it increases glucose utilization and also suppresses hepatic glucose production, IGF-1 has a hypoglycemic potential. To reduce the risk of hypoglycemia, it should be administered (twice a day) within 20 minutes before or after a meal or a snack.

Mecasermin rinfabate (Iplex – Insmed)
Agent for Growth Failure
2006 (no longer marketed)

New Drug Comparison Rating (NDCR) =4 (significant advantages).

Indication:

Administered subcutaneously for the treatment of growth failure in children with severe primary insulin-like growth factor-1 (IGF-1) deficiency or with growth hormone gene deletion who have developed neutralizing antibodies to growth hormone.

Comparable drugs:

Mecasermin (Increlex).

Advantages:

- Administered once a day (compared with twice a day with mecasermin).
- More flexibility in administration (does not have to be administered in close proximity to a meal or snack).

Disadvantages:

- Must be stored in a frozen state.
- Available only through a restricted distribution program (marketing has been subsequently discontinued).

Most important risks/adverse events:

Contraindicated in patients with closed epiphyses, and in the presence of active or suspected neoplasia; hypoglycemia; local or systemic allergic reactions; lymphoid tissue (e.g., tonsillar) hypertrophy; intracranial hypertension; slipped capital femoral epiphysis; worsening of scoliosis.

Most common adverse events:

Hypoglycemia (31%), headache (22%), tonsillar and/or adenoid hypertrophy (19%), and the following adverse events in at least 5% of patients—arthralgia, bone pain, pain in an extremity, muscular atrophy, papilledema, hematuria, ovarian cysts, iron deficiency anemia, lymphadenopathy, thyromegaly, injection site reactions, and increased transaminases.

Usual dosage:

Administered subcutaneously once a day in the morning or in the evening but at approximately the same time each day; recommended initial dosage is 0.5 mg/kg once a day, and the dosage can be titrated up to a maximum of 2 mg/kg once a day.

Product:

Vials – 36 mg (must be stored frozen while in the distribution chain).

Comments:

In the circulation, more than 80% of IGF-1 is bound as a complex with IGF-binding protein-3 (IGFBP-3) and an acid-labile subunit. Mecasermin rinfabate contains recombinant IGF-1 in the form of a binary protein complex with IGFBP-3 that is also produced using recombinant technology. The binding protein does not have a growth-promoting effect, but it extends the time that IGF-1 remains in the blood, thereby permitting once-daily administration.

Mecasermin rinfabate and mecasermin have not been directly compared in clinical studies. The FDA first approved mecasermin and subsequently approved mecasermin rinfabate. Because of patent issues and other considerations, mecasermin rinfabate is no longer marketed.

Methylnaltrexone bromide (Relistor – Progenics; Wyeth)
Agent for Opioid-Induced Constipation
2008

New Drug Comparison Rating (NDCR) = 4 (significant advantages)

Indication:

Administered subcutaneously for the treatment of opioid-induced constipation in patients with advanced illness who are receiving palliative care, when the response to laxative therapy has not been sufficient.

Comparable drugs:

Laxatives (e.g., senna [e.g., Senokot]), stool softeners (e.g., docusate [e.g., Colace]).

Advantages:

- Is often effective in relieving opioid-induced constipation in patients whose response to laxatives has not been sufficient.
- Has a unique mechanism of action for the treatment of opioid-induced constipation.

Disadvantages:

- Must be administered by injection (subcutaneously).
- May be more likely to cause gastrointestinal adverse events.

Most important risks/adverse events:

Contraindicated in patients with known or suspected mechanical gastrointestinal obstruction; if severe or persistent diarrhea occurs during treatment, the drug should be discontinued; dosage should be reduced in patients with severe renal impairment; if the opioid analgesic is discontinued, the use of methylnaltrexone should also be discontinued.

Most common adverse events:

Abdominal pain (29%), flatulence (13%), nausea (12%), dizziness (7%), diarrhea (6%).

Usual dosage:

Administered subcutaneously and the usual frequency of administration is one dose every other day as needed; no more than one dose should be administered in a 24-hour period; recommended dose is 8 mg for patients weighing 38-61 kg (84-135 pounds), and 12 mg for patients weighing 62-114 kg (136-251 pounds); for patients weighing less than 38 kg or more than 114 kg, a dosage of 0.15 mg/kg should be used; in patients with severe renal impairment (creatinine clearance less than 30 mL/minute), the dosage should be reduced by one-half.

Product:

Vials – 12 mg (in 0.6 mL of solution); should be kept away from light.

Comments:

Opioid analgesics such as morphine are often used on a continuous basis to relieve pain associated with incurable cancers and other advanced illnesses. In addition to acting at opioid receptors in the central nervous system to provide their analgesic action, the opioid analgesics also act at opioid receptors in peripheral receptors in the gastrointestinal tract, one of the consequences of which is that almost all patients who are treated with these analgesics on a continuous basis will experience constipation. To reduce the likelihood of constipation, the use of a bowel regimen (e.g., laxatives, stool softeners) is usually recommended for patients who are to be treated with an opioid analgesic on a regular basis. For many patients, however, even the use of a bowel regimen is insufficient to prevent opioid-induced constipation.

Methylnaltrexone is an opioid antagonist that is related to naltrexone (e.g., ReVia, Vivitrol) that has been used for the treatment of alcohol and opioid dependence. However, methylnaltrexone does not cross the blood-brain barrier and it functions as a selective peripherally-acting mu-opioid receptor antagonist in tissues such as the gastrointestinal tract. Therefore, it decreases the constipating action of opioid analgesics without reducing the centrally-mediated analgesic effects. The effectiveness of methylnaltrexone was demonstrated in placebo-controlled studies. In a single-dose study, approximately 60% of the patients experienced a laxative action within 4 hours following administration, compared with 14% of those receiving placebo. When administered every other day, those receiving the drug had a higher rate of laxation within 4 hours of the first dose (48%) than placebo-treated patients (16%).

Micafungin sodium (Mycamine – Astellas)
Antifungal Agent
2005

New Drug Comparison Rating (NDCR) = 3 (no or minor advantages/disadvantages)

Indications:
Administered via intravenous infusion for the treatment of esophageal candidiasis, and for prophylaxis of Candida infections in patients undergoing hematopoietic stem cell transplantation; (has been subsequently approved for the treatment of patients with candidemia, acute disseminated candidiasis, Candida peritonitis and abscesses).

Comparable drugs:
Caspofungin (Cancidas); (another comparable drug, anidulafungin [Eraxis] was marketed in 2006).

Advantages:
- Has a labeled indication for prophylaxis against Candida infections.
- Is not likely to interact with cyclosporine.

Disadvantages:
- Has fewer labeled indications (has subsequently been approved for additional indications).
- May be more likely to cause hypersensitivity reactions.

Most important risks/adverse events:
Hypersensitivity reactions; liver function test abnormalities.

Most common adverse events:
Nausea (3%), vomiting (2%), headache (2%), elevations of ALT (3%) and AST (3%).

Usual dosage:
Esophageal candidiasis – 150 mg once a day via intravenous infusion over a period of 1 hour; prophylaxis of Candida infections – 50 mg once a day via intravenous infusion over a period of 1 hour; other labeled indications – 100 mg once a day via intravenous infusion over a period of 1 hour.

Products:
Vials – 50 mg, 100 mg.

Comments:

Micafungin is the second echinocandin antifungal agent marketed in the United States, joining caspofungin (A third agent, anidulafungin [Eraxis] joined this class in 2006.) These agents inhibit the synthesis of a glucan derivative that is an essential component of fungal cell walls but not present in mammalian cells. They are administered via intravenous infusion and, unlike many of the azole antifungal agents, are not available in orally administered formulations.

Micafungin was compared with the intravenous use of fluconazole (e.g., Diflucan) in the clinical studies, and the efficacy results were similar for the two agents. The labeled indications for micafungin are much more limited than those for caspofungin. (However, additional indications for micafungin have subsequently been approved.) The indications for caspofungin include treatment of esophageal candidiasis, candidemia, and intra-abdominal abscesses, peritonitis, and pleural space infections caused by Candida, invasive aspergillosis in patients who are refractory to or intolerant of other antifungal therapy, and empirical therapy for presumed fungal infections in febrile neutropenic patients..

Micafungin does not interact with cyclosporine (e.g., Neoral) which is an advantage over caspofungin, for which there is a warning regarding elevations of hepatic enzymes with concurrent use.

Milnacipran hydrochloride (Savella – Forest; Cypress)
Agent for Fibromyalgia
2009

New Drug Comparison Rating (NDCR) = 3 (no or minor advantages/disadvantages)

Indication:
Management of fibromyalgia.

Comparable drugs:
Duloxetine (Cymbalta), pregabalin (Lyrica).

Advantages:
- Is a more potent inhibitor of norepinephrine reuptake than serotonin reuptake that may be advantageous in some patients (compared with duloxetine).
- Is not a controlled substance (compared with pregabalin that is in Schedule V).
- Less likely to interact with other medications (e.g., CYP1A2 inhibitors, CYP2D6 inhibitors) via pharmacokinetic mechanisms (compared with duloxetine that is a substrate for these metabolic pathways).
- Less likely to cause hypersensitivity reactions and angioedema, edema and weight gain, and creatine kinase elevations (compared with pregabalin).
- May be used (in reduced dosage) in patients with severe renal impairment (compared with duloxetine).
- May be used (with caution) in patients with hepatic impairment (compared with duloxetine).

Disadvantages:
- Fewer labeled indications (duloxetine is also indicated for the acute and maintenance treatment of major depressive disorder, the acute treatment of generalized anxiety disorder, and for the management of neuropathic pain associated with diabetic peripheral neuropathy; pregabalin is also indicated for the management of neuropathic pain associated with diabetic peripheral neuropathy, the management of postherpetic neuralgia, and as adjunctive therapy for adult patients with partial onset seizures).
- Dosage titration is more complex (compared with duloxetine for which just one dosage adjustment is recommended).
- More contraindications (i.e., interactions with monoamine oxidase inhibitors [MAOIs], patients with uncontrolled narrow-angle glaucoma) (compared with pregabalin).
- Greater risk of hepatic adverse events (compared with pregabalin).
- More likely to cause increased blood pressure and heart rate, serotonin syndrome, abnormal bleeding, nausea, and urinary hesitancy/retention (compared with pregabalin).

Most important risks/adverse events:
Risk of suicidal thinking and behavior in children, adolescents, and young adults (boxed warning [is not indicated for use in pediatric patients]); contraindicated in patients being treated with an MAOI or within 14 days of discontinuing treatment with an MAOI; treatment with an MAOI should not be initiated for at least 5 days following discontinuation of treatment with milnacipran; use is contraindicated in patients with uncontrolled narrow-angle glaucoma; serotonin syndrome

(risk is greater in patients who are also treated with other drugs that may affect serotonergic systems [e.g., selective serotonin reuptake inhibitors {SSRIs}, serotonin and norepinephrine reuptake inhibitors {SNRIs}, triptans, tramadol {e.g., Ultram}], or drugs that impair metabolism of serotonin [MAOIs]); elevated blood pressure and heart rate (should be determined prior to initiating treatment and periodically during treatment); hepatotoxicity (should not ordinarily be prescribed for patients with substantial alcohol use or evidence of chronic liver disease); abnormal bleeding (risk is increased in patients also taking an anticoagulant, aspirin, or anti-inflammatory drug); activation of mania; hyponatremia; may affect urethral resistance and micturition (risk is greater in men with benign prostatic hyperplasia); Pregnancy Category C; patients should be advised to avoid consuming alcoholic beverages.

Most common adverse events:

Nausea (35%), constipation (16%), dizziness (11%), hot flush (11%), hyperhidrosis (8%), palpitations (8%), hypertension (7%), vomiting (6%), dry mouth (5%), increased heart rate (5%), headache (19%, but at a similar incidence with placebo).

Usual dosage:

recommended maintenance dosage is 50 mg twice a day; treatment is initiated with a single dose of 12.5 mg on the first day, followed by 12.5 mg twice a day on days 2 and 3, 25 mg twice a day on days 4 through 7, and 50 mg twice a day thereafter; dosage may be increased to 100 mg twice a day based on individual patient response; in patients with severe renal impairment, the usual maintenance dosage should be reduced to 25 mg twice a day; treatment should not be abruptly discontinued following extended use, but rather the dosage should be gradually reduced.

Products:

Tablets – 12.5 mg, 25 mg, 50 mg, 100 mg.

Comments:

Fibromyalgia typically develops in early-to-middle adulthood, and is most often experienced by women. The most common symptoms are muscle soreness and tenderness, flu-like aching, dull pain in the muscles, morning stiffness, fatigue, and problems sleeping. The American College of Rheumatology has identified criteria for a diagnosis of fibromyalgia that include widespread pain that lasts for at least 3 months, plus pain present at 11 or more of the 18 parts of the body called "tender points."

Milnacipran (Savella) is the third drug to be approved for the management of fibromyalgia, joining pregabalin and duloxetine. Like duloxetine, venlafaxine (e.g., Effexor XR), and desvenlafaxine (Pristiq), the new drug is a serotonin and norepinephrine reuptake inhibitor (SNRI). Milnacipran is a racemic mixture and its active enantiomer, d-milnacipran, inhibits norepinephrine uptake with approximately 3-fold higher potency in vitro than serotonin uptake. Its effectiveness in the management of fibromyalgia was demonstrated in two placebo-controlled studies in which a larger proportion of the patients treated with the drug experienced a simultaneous reduction in pain from baseline of at least 30% and also rated themselves as much improved or very much improved based on a patient global assessment. In addition, a larger proportion of patients treated with milnacipran met the criteria for treatment response, as measured by the composite endpoint that concurrently evaluated improvement in pain, physical function, and patient global assessment.

The drug-related problems, warnings, and precautions associated with the use of milnacipran are generally similar to those of duloxetine and the other SNRIs, as well as the SSRIs. However, unlike duloxetine, milnacipran undergoes minimal metabolism via cytochrome P450 pathways, and is less likely to interact with other medications via pharmacokinetic mechanisms. In the clinical studies, 23% of the patients discontinued treatment prematurely due to adverse events, compared with 12% of those receiving placebo.

Nebivolol hydrochloride (Bystolic – Forest)
Antihypertensive Agent
2008

New Drug Comparison Rating (NDCR) = 3 (no or minor advantages/disadvantages)

Indication:

Treatment of hypertension; may be used alone or in combination with other antihypertensive agents.

Comparable drug:

Carvedilol (Coreg).

Advantages:

- Less risk in patients with asthma or related bronchospastic conditions (carvedilol is contraindicated).
- May increase nitric oxide-mediated vasodilatation.

Disadvantages:

- Indications are limited (carvedilol is also indicated in patients with heart failure and in patients with left ventricular dysfunction following myocardial infarction).
- Dosage should be reduced in patients with severe renal impairment or moderate hepatic impairment.

Most important risks/adverse events:

Contraindicated in patients with severe bradycardia, heart block greater than first degree, cardiogenic shock, decompensated heart failure, sick sinus syndrome (unless a permanent pacemaker is in place), or severe hepatic impairment; should generally be avoided in patients with bronchospastic diseases, although risk is lower than with the nonselective beta-blockers); may mask some of the manifestations of hypoglycemia, particularly tachycardia; may mask clinical signs of hyperthyroidism (e.g., tachycardia); may precipitate or aggravate symptoms in patients with peripheral vascular disease; patients with a history of severe anaphylactic reactions may be more reactive to subsequent exposure to the allergen and less responsive to usual doses of epinephrine used to treat allergic reaction; is a substrate of CYP2D6 and action may be increased by the concurrent use of a CYP2D6 inhibitor (e.g., fluoxetine [e.g., Prozac]); increased risk of cardiovascular adverse events when used concurrently with digoxin, diltiazem (e.g., Cardizem), or verapamil (e.g., Covera-HS).

Most common adverse events (incidences reported with a dosage of 10 mg daily):

Headache (6%), dizziness (3%), nausea (3%), diarrhea (2%), fatigue (2%).

Usual dosage:

5 mg once a day initially, as monotherapy or in combination with other antihypertensive agents; if needed, dosage may be increased at 2-week intervals up to 40 mg once a day; in patients with severe renal impairment or moderate hepatic impairment, the recommended initial dosage is 2.5 mg once a day; if a dose is missed, patient should take the next dose at the scheduled time; if treatment is to be discontinued, should taper over 1 to 2 weeks.

Products:

Tablets – 2.5 mg, 5 mg, 10 mg.

Comments:

Nebivolol is a preferentially $beta_1$-selective (cardioselective) beta-adrenergic blocking agent (beta-blocker) when used in doses of 10 mg or less in patients who are extensive metabolizers of the drug (most of the population). However, it inhibits both $beta_1$ and $beta_2$ receptors at higher doses and in patients who are poor metabolizers. It has been suggested to reduce vascular resistance by increasing nitric oxide-mediated vasodilatation although specific clinical and safety benefits attributable to this action have not been conclusively demonstrated. Unlike carvedilol, it does not inhibit $alpha_1$-adrenergic receptors and it does not have labeled indications for the treatment of patients with heart failure or patients with left ventricular dysfunction following myocardial infarction.

Nebivolol is a racemic mixture that is composed of d- and l-isomers. Although the exposure to l-nebivolol is higher than for d-nebivolol, the l-isomer contributes little to the drug's activity as the beta receptor affinity of the active d-isomer is more than 1000-fold higher than that for the l-isomer. The new drug is primarily metabolized via direct glucuronidation and to a lesser extent via N-dealkylation and oxidation via CYP2D6. Its concentration and activity may be increased by the concurrent use of a CYP2D6 inhibitor (e.g., fluoxetine).

Nelarabine (Arranon – GlaxoSmithKline)
Antineoplastic Agent
2006

New Drug Comparison Rating (NDCR) = 5 (important advance)

Indications:

Administered via intravenous infusion for the treatment of patients with T-cell acute lymphoblastic leukemia (T-ALL) and T-cell lymphoblastic lymphoma (T-LBL) whose disease has not responded to or has relapsed following treatment with at least two chemotherapy regimens.

Comparable drugs (for use in treating ALL):

e.g., cytarabine (e.g., Cytosar-U), doxorubicin (e.g., Adriamycin), asparaginase (Elspar), pegaspargase (Oncaspar), mercaptopurine (e.g., Purinethol), methotrexate (e.g., Trexall), teniposide (Vumon), vincristine (e.g., Vincasar), clofarabine (Clolar).

Advantages:

- First drug to be approved for the treatment of T-ALL and T-LBL.
- May be effective in some patients who are refractory to or who have relapsed with other treatment.

Disadvantages:

- Not approved for first-line treatment.
- Clinical benefit (e.g., prolonged survival) has not yet been demonstrated.
- May cause neurotoxicity.

Most important risks/adverse events:

Neurologic events (boxed warning – e.g., altered mental status, seizures, peripheral neuropathy); hematologic events (e.g., neutropenia, anemia, thrombocytopenia – complete blood counts including platelets should be monitored regularly); tumor lysis syndrome (intravenous hydration should be provided); may cause harm to a fetus and should not be used during pregnancy.

Most common adverse events:

In pediatric patients – headache (17%), peripheral neurologic disorders (12%), vomiting (10%), anemia (95%), neutropenia (94%), thrombocytopenia (88%); in adult patients – fatigue (50%), nausea (41%), somnolence (23%), dizziness (21%), peripheral neurologic disorders (21%), pyrexia (23%), diarrhea (22%), vomiting (22%), constipation (21%), asthenia (17%), hypoesthesia (17%), headache (15%), anemia (99%), thrombocytopenia (86%), neutropenia (81%).

Usual dosage:

Administered as an intravenous infusion; in adult patients – 1,500 mg/m^2 as a 2-hour infusion on days 1, 3, and 5 repeated every 21 days; in pediatric patients – 650 mg/m^2 as a 1-hour infusion for 5 consecutive days every 21 days.

Product:

Vials – 250 mg.

Comments:

Acute lymphoblastic leukemia (ALL) is the most common form of pediatric leukemia and approximately 20% of those afflicted have a form of the disease designated as T-cell ALL (T-ALL). Lymphoblastic lymphoma (LBL) is responsible for approximately 30% of childhood and 3% of adult non-Hodgkin's lymphoma (NHL). Of the approximately 50,000 patients who are diagnosed with NHL each year, an estimated 900 have T-cell LBL (T-LBL). Nelarabine is the first drug to be approved for the treatment of T-ALL and T-LBL and is indicated for patients whose disease has not responded to or has relapsed following treatment with at least two chemotherapy regimens. It was approved using the FDA's accelerated approval process based on the induction of complete responses; clinical benefit (e.g., prolonged survival) has not yet been demonstrated. Clinical studies of nelarabine were conducted in both pediatric (21 years and younger) and adult patients, and complete responses were experienced in 23% and 21% of these groups of patients, respectively.

Nelarabine is a prodrug of the cytotoxic deoxyguanosine analogue, 9-beta-d-arabinofuranosylguanine (ara-G), and is rapidly converted to ara-G following intravenous administration. Ara-G is subsequently converted to its active triphosphate metabolite, ara-GTP, that accumulates in leukemic blasts and is incorporated into DNA, resulting in inhibition of DNA synthesis and cell death.

Nepafenac (Nevanac – Alcon)
Anti-inflammatory Drug
2005

New Drug Comparison Rating (NDCR) = 4 (significant advantages)

Indication:

For ophthalmic administration for the treatment of pain and inflammation associated with cataract surgery.

Comparable drugs:

Ophthalmic NSAIDs—Bromfenac (Xibrom), diclofenac (Voltaren), ketorolac (Acular).

Advantages:

- Labeled indication includes treatment of pain and inflammation (other agents are indicated for inflammation associated with cataract surgery).
- May attain greater ocular penetration.
- May cause less burning and stinging (compared with diclofenac and ketorolac).
- Administered less frequently (compared with diclofenac and ketorolac, which are administered four times a day).

Disadvantages:

- Has fewer ophthalmic labeled indications (compared with diclofenac and ketorolac).
- Administered more frequently (compared with bromfenac, which is administered twice a day).

Most important risks/adverse events:

Potential for cross-sensitivity in patients with a history of hypersensitivity to a nonsteroidal anti-inflammatory drug (NSAID) or aspirin; increased bleeding time.

Most common adverse events:

Ocular adverse events (possibly attributable to the surgical procedure and not the medication) occurring in 5% to 10% of patients – capsular opacity, decreased visual acuity, foreign body sensation, increased intraocular pressure.

Usual dosage:

One drop in the affected eye(s) 3 times a day beginning 1 day prior to cataract surgery, continued on the day of surgery and through the first 2 weeks of the postoperative period.

Product:

Ophthalmic suspension – 0.1%.

Comments:

Nepafenac is a nonsteroidal anti-inflammatory prodrug for ophthalmic use. Following ophthalmic administration, nepafenac penetrates the cornea and is converted by ocular tissue hydrolases to amfenac, a potent inhibitor of cyclooxygenases. Nepafenac may attain greater penetration into ocular tissue than other NSAIDs; however, it has not been directly compared with the other agents.

Bromfenac, diclofenac, and ketorolac are indicated for the treatment of postoperative inflammation following cataract extraction and nepafenac is the only NSAID approved for both pain and inflammation associated with cataract surgery. Treatment with nepafenac is initiated 1 day prior to surgery whereas treatment with the other agents is initiated 24 hours after surgery.

Nilotinib (Tasigna – Novartis)
Antineoplastic Agent
2007

New Drug Comparison Rating (NDCR) = 3 (no or minor advantages/disadvantages)

Indication:
Treatment of chronic phase and accelerated phase Philadelphia chromosome positive chronic myelogenous leukemia (CML) in adult patients resistant to or intolerant to prior therapy that included imatinib (Gleevec).

Comparable drugs:
Imatinib (Gleevec), dasatinib (Sprycel).

Advantages:
• May be effective in some patients who are no longer responding to, or who can no longer tolerate, other therapies.

Disadvantages:
• Is not indicated for first-line treatment (compared with imatinib).
• Labeled indications are more limited (dasatinib is also indicated for certain types of acute lymphoblastic leukemia and imatinib has numerous other indications including the treatment of patients with gastrointestinal stromal tumors).
• May be more likely to cause QT interval prolongation.
• Administered twice a day (compared with once a day for the comparable drugs).

Most important risks/adverse events:
QT interval prolongation (boxed warning; use is contraindicated in patients with hypokalemia, hypomagnesemia, or long QT syndrome; concurrent use of drugs that prolong the QT interval [e.g., antiarrhythmic agents, moxifloxacin (Avelox)] or strong CYP3A4 inhibitors [e.g., clarithromycin (e.g., Biaxin), grapefruit products] should be avoided; food increases concentration and should be avoided for 2 hours before and 1 hour after each dose; electrocardiograms should be obtained at baseline, 7 days after initiating treatment, and periodically thereafter); myelosuppression (neutropenia, thrombocytopenia, anemia; complete blood counts should be done every 2 weeks for the first 2 months, then monthly); ventricular repolarization abnormalities; electrolyte abnormalities (electrolytes should be periodically monitored); liver function abnormality (e.g., elevations in ALT, AST, bilirubin; liver function tests should be performed periodically); elevated serum lipase (patients with a history of pancreatitis should be closely monitored); may cause harm to a fetus and should not be used during pregnancy.

133

Most common adverse events (and the incidences reported in the studies in patients with chronic phase CML):

Grade 3 or 4 thrombocytopenia (28%), grade 3 or 4 neutropenia (28%), rash (33%), pruritus (29%), headache (31%), nausea (31%), fatigue (28%), diarrhea (22%), constipation (21%), vomiting (21%).

Usual dosage:

400 mg twice a day, approximately 12 hours apart, at least 2 hours before and at least one hour after food; capsules should be swallowed whole with water.

Product:

Capsules -200 mg.

Comments:

Many patients with chronic myeloid leukemia (CML) have experienced the formation of an abnormal fusion protein known as BCR-ABL that has enhanced activity as a tyrosine kinase, and is associated with uncontrolled proliferation of abnormal white blood cells. Imatinib blocks the BCR-ABL tyrosine kinase and is often considered the first-line treatment. However, some patients have experienced resistance or serious adverse events that preclude the continuation of imatinib treatment. Nilotinib is a kinase inhibitor that inhibits the BCR-ABL kinase. In studies in patients with chronic phase CML (CML-CP) who were imatinib –resistant or intolerant, the use of nilotinib provided a cytogenetic response rate of 40% (28% complete response; 12% partial response). In patients with accelerated phase CML (CML-AP) treated with nilotinib, the hematologic response rate was 26% (18% complete response; 8% partial response). These studies are continuing but 59% of CML-CP patients with a major cytogenetic response and 63% of CML-AP patients with a hematologic response had a duration of response of at least 6 months.

Ofatumumab (Arzerra – GlaxoSmithKline)
Antineoplastic Agent
2009

New Drug Comparison Rating (NDCR) = 4 (significant advantages)

Indication:

Administered via intravenous infusion for the treatment of patients with chronic lymphocytic leukemia (CLL) refractory to fludarabine and alemtuzumab.

Comparable drugs:

Fludarabine (e.g., Fludara, Oforta), alemtuzumab (Campath), rituximab (Rituxan).

Advantages:

- Effective in some patients who are refractory to fludarabine and alemtuzumab.
- Has a labeled indication for chronic lymphocytic leukemia (compared with rituximab that does not have this labeled indication; however, it is often used as a first-line treatment for CLL).
- Better tolerated by some patients.

Disadvantages:

- Not indicated as a first-line treatment.
- Has not been directly compared with rituximab in clinical studies.
- Fewer labeled indications (compared with rituximab that has indications for non-Hodgkin's lymphoma and rheumatoid arthritis).
- Recommended doses require use of multiple vials (e.g., 20 vials for a dose of 2,000 mg).

Most important risks/adverse events:

Serious infusion reactions (e.g., bronchospasm, dyspnea, laryngeal edema, syncope, pyrexia, urticaria, angioedema; reactions occur more frequently with the first 2 infusions; patients should be premedicated with acetaminophen, an antihistamine, and a corticosteroid); cytopenias (e.g., neutropenia, thrombocytopenia; complete blood counts and platelet counts should be monitored at regular intervals); progressive multifocal leukoencephalopathy (PML); hepatitis B reactivation; intestinal obstruction; administration of live vaccines should be avoided.

Most common adverse events:

Neutropenia (42% with Grade 3 or 4 severity), infusion reactions (44% on the day of the first infusion, and less frequently during subsequent infusions), pneumonia (23%), pyrexia (20%), cough (19%), diarrhea (18%), anemia (16%), fatigue (15%), dyspnea (14%), rash (14%), upper respiratory tract infection (11%), bronchitis (11%), nausea (11%).

Usual dosage:

Administered via intravenous infusion with an in-line filter supplied with the product (must not be administered via push or bolus); patients should be premedicated 30 minutes to 2 hours prior to each dose (e.g., with acetaminophen, an antihistamine, and intravenous corticosteroid); an initial dose of 300 mg (dose 1) is followed 1 week later by 2,000 mg weekly for 7 doses (doses 2 through 8), followed 4 weeks later by 2,000 mg every 4 weeks for 4 doses (doses 9 through 12); different infusion rates are recommended for dose 1, dose 2, and doses 3 through 12; infusion should be interrupted if infusion reactions occur.

Product:

Single-use vials – 100 mg/5 mL; should be stored in a refrigerator; doses should be prepared in 1,000 mL of 0.9% Sodium Chloride Injection.

Comments:

Chronic lymphocytic leukemia is a slowly progressing cancer of the blood and bone marrow that primarily affects people older than 50. Antineoplastic agents that have been used in the treatment of CLL include chlorambucil (e.g., Leukeran), fludarabine, alemtuzumab, bendamustine (Treanda), cyclophosphamide, and rituximab. CLL is not yet a labeled indication for rituximab but this agent is often included in first-line regimens for this condition.

The CD20 molecule is expressed on the surface of normal B lymphocytes and on malignant B-cells in patients with CLL. Ofatumumab is a human monoclonal antibody that binds to the CD20 antigen, as does rituximab, although there are distinctions in the nature of the binding of the two agents to CD20. The effectiveness of the new drug was demonstrated in a study in which 42% of patients with CLL who were refractory to both fludarabine and alemtuzumab responded to treatment with ofatumumab. These patients had a median duration of response of 6.5 months.

Omega-3-acid ethyl esters (Lovaza* – GlaxoSmithKline)
Lipid-Regulating Agent
2005

New Drug Comparison Rating (NDCR) = 4 (significant advantages)

Indication:
Adjunct to diet to reduce very high (at least 500 mg/dL) triglyceride concentrations in adult patients.

Comparable drugs:
Fenofibrate (e.g., Tricor), gemfibrozil (e.g., Lopid), dietary supplements containing EPA and DHA omega-3 fatty acids.

Advantages:
- Unique mechanism of action (compared with the fibrates).
- Less likely to cause adverse events and interact with other medications (compared with the fibrates).
- Clinical effectiveness has been demonstrated and an effective dosage identified (compared with dietary supplements).

Disadvantages:
- More likely to cause taste perversion and eructation (compared with the fibrates).

Most important risks/adverse events:
May prolong bleeding time and caution should be exercised in patients being treated with an anticoagulant; should be used with caution in patients who are allergic to fish.

Most common adverse events:
Eructation (4%), taste perversion (3%), flu syndrome (3%), infection (3%).

Usual dosage:
Four grams a day administered as a single 4-gram dose or as two 2-gram doses.

Product:
Capsules – 1 gram (containing at least 900 mg of the ethyl esters of omega-3 fatty acids, which are predominantly a combination of ethyl esters of eicosapentaenoic acid {EPA, approximately 465 mg] and docosahexaenoic acid [DHA, approximately 375 mg]).

Comments:

Omega-3 fatty acids are long-chained, polyunsaturated fatty acids that have been suggested to be of value in reducing the risk of certain cardiovascular problems and in the treatment of certain other clinical problems. The body cannot synthesize these fatty acids so they must be supplied via dietary sources (e.g., oily fish) or in the form of supplements or therapeutic agents. The most extensively studied of these fatty acids are eicosapentaenoic acid (EPA) and docosahexaenoic acid (DHA) omega-3 fatty acids.

Omega-3-acid ethyl esters is the first product containing omega-3 fatty acids to be approved by the FDA. In placebo-controlled studies, it reduced triglyceride concentrations by as much as 50%. The product is safer than the fibrates and provides an additional option to reduce very high triglyceride concentrations. In patients with combined dyslipidemias (e.g., those with both hypercholesterolemia and hypertriglyceridemia) that are not adequately controlled with the use of a statin (e.g., atorvastatin [Lipitor]) alone, the combined use of a statin with omega-3-acid ethyl esters (rather than a fibrate) may provide a safer combination regimen.

*Omacor was the trade name under which the product was initially marketed. However, because of mistakes resulting from the similarity of this name to that of Amicar, the trade name for the omega-3-acid ethyl esters product was changed to Lovaza in 2007.

Palifermin (Kepivance – Amgen)
Agent for Oral Mucositis
2005

New Drug Comparison Rating (NDCR) = 5 (important advance)

Indication:
Administered intravenously to decrease the incidence and duration of severe oral mucositis in patients with hematologic malignancies receiving myelotoxic therapy requiring hematopoietic stem cell support.

Comparable drugs:
None.

Advantages:
• First drug approved for the treatment of severe oral mucositis.

Disadvantages/Limitations:
• Must be administered intravenously.
• Available only through a restricted distribution program.

Most important risks/adverse events:
Potential for stimulation of tumor growth in patients with nonhematologic malignancies.

Most common adverse events:
Rash (62%, compared with 50% in the placebo group), pruritus (35%), erythema (32%), mouth/tongue thickness or discoloration (17%), altered taste (16%), arthralgia (10%).

Usual dosage:
60 mcg/kg/day administered as an intravenous bolus injection for 3 consecutive days before and 3 consecutive days after myelotoxic therapy for a total of 6 doses; the last dose of the first series of 3 doses should be administered 24 to 48 hours before myelotoxic therapy; the second series of 3 doses should be administered following myelotoxic therapy; the first of these doses should be administered after, but on the same day of hematopoietic stem cell infusion and at least 4 days after the most recent administration of palifermin.

Product:
Vials – 6.25 mg (should be stored in a refrigerator).

Comments:

Almost all patients with hematologic malignancies (e.g., Hodgkin's disease, non-Hodgkin's lymphoma, leukemias, multiple myeloma) who undergo bone marrow transplantation experience the complication of oral mucositis. Severe oral mucositis is characterized by the development of sores and ulcers in the lining of the mouth, resulting in severe pain and difficulty eating, drinking, swallowing, and talking. Palifermin is the first drug to be developed for the management of oral mucositis. It is a modified form of human keratinocyte growth factor (KGF) that is produced using recombinant DNA technology. KGF is a naturally occurring human protein that stimulates the growth of cells in the surface layer of the mouth as well as in other tissues. Like the natural KGF, palifermin binds to KGF receptors and stimulates cell reproduction, growth, and development, resulting in faster replacement of the cells killed by chemotherapy and radiation therapy, and increasing the rate of healing.

In a study of patients with leukemia or lymphoma treated with high doses of chemotherapy and radiation in conjunction with bone marrow transplantation, 98% of those who did not receive palifermin developed severe oral mucositis compared to 63% of those who received the drug. In addition, severe mucositis lasted an average of only 3 days in those receiving palifermin compared to 9 days for those not receiving the drug. Thus, the new drug represents an important advance for the management of a serious complication for which no specific treatment was previously available.

Paliperidone (Invega – Janssen)
Antipsychotic Agent
2007

New Drug Comparison Rating (NDCR) = 2 (significant disadvantages)

Indication:

Acute and maintenance treatment of schizophrenia (subsequently approved for the acute treatment of schizoaffective disorder as monotherapy, and as an adjunct to mood stabilizers and/or antidepressants; in addition, an extended-release parenteral formulation of paliperidone palmitate [Invega Sustenna] has been approved for the treatment of schizophrenia).

Comparable drug:

Risperidone (Risperdal).

Advantages:

- Dosage titration usually not necessary.
- Less risk of interactions with CYP2D6 inducers (e.g., carbamazepine [e.g., Tegretol]).
- Less potential for variation in response in patients with low CYP2D6 activity.
- First drug for schizophrenia for which information regarding the Personal and Social Performance (PSP) evaluation is included in the labeling.

Disadvantages:

- Has not been directly compared with risperidone in clinical studies.
- Indication for schizophrenia is more limited (risperidone has also been demonstrated to prevent relapses).
- Fewer labeled indications (risperidone is also indicated for the short-term treatment of acute manic or mixed episodes associated with Bipolar I Disorder, and for the treatment of irritability associated with autistic disorder in children and adolescents [ages 5 to 18]).
- May cause QT interval prolongation.
- Restrictions regarding use in patients with gastrointestinal (GI) disorders that may impede GI transit of tablet formulation.
- No/limited experience in pediatric patients.
- Fewer formulation options (risperidone is also available as an oral solution, orally disintegrating tablets, and in a long-acting parenteral formulation for intramuscular administration).

Most important risks/adverse events:

Increased mortality in elderly patients with dementia-related psychosis (boxed warning; is not approved for the treatment of patients with dementia-related psychosis); QT interval prolongation (should not be used in patients at risk including those taking other medications that are known to cause QT prolongation [e.g., certain antiarrhythmic agents, moxifloxacin {Avelox}]); neuroleptic malignant syndrome; tardive dyskinesia; hyperglycemia/diabetes mellitus; cerebrovascular adverse events; GI obstructive symptoms (extended-release tablet formulation is swallowed whole and the tablet shell remains intact during GI transit; should not be used in patients with pre-existing severe GI narrowing or other conditions that would restrict/limit transit of the tablet); cognitive and motor impairment; orthostatic hypotension/syncope; seizures; hyperprolactinemia; dysphagia; priapism; thrombotic thrombocytopenic purpura; disruption of body temperature regulation; suicide (risk inherent in psychiatric illness); may reduce the action of levodopa and other dopamine agonists (a warning about leukopenia, neutropenia, and agranulocytosis has been subequently added to the labeling).

Most common adverse events (and the incidence reported with the usual dosage of 6 mg once a day):

Tachycardia (12%), headache (12%), somnolence (9%), weight gain (6%), QT interval prolongation (4%), akathisia (3%), extrapyramidal disorder (2%).

Usual dosage:

6 mg once a day in the morning with the aid of liquids; dosage may be increased in increments of 3 mg/day at intervals of more than 5 days to the maximum recommended dosage of 12 mg once a day; dosage should be reduced in patients with renal impairment.

Products:

Extended-release tablets – 3 mg, 6 mg, 9 mg (1.5 mg tablets have been subequently marketed; has also been marketed in an extended-release parenteral formulation [Invega Sustenna] in 39 mg, 78 mg, 117 mg, 156 mg, and 234 mg potencies).

Comments:

Paliperidone is the major active metabolite of risperidone but has not been directly compared with its parent compound in clinical trials. They are thought to exhibit their antipsychotic activity through a combination of central dopamine type 2 (D2) and serotonin type 2 (5-HT2A) receptor antagonism. The labeled indications for, and available formulations of, paliperidone are much more limited than those for risperidone. Patients should be advised that the tablets should be swallowed whole.

Panitumumab (Vectibix — Amgen)
Antineoplastic Agent
2006

New Drug Comparison Rating (NDCR) = 4 (significant advantages)

Indication:

Administered via intravenous infusion for the treatment of epidermal growth factor receptors (EGFR)-expressing metastatic colorectal carcinoma with disease progression on or following fluoropyrimidine-, oxaliplatin-, and irinotecan-containing chemotherapy regimens (subsequently revised to add a notation that use is not recommended in patients whose tumors had KRAS mutations in codon 12 or 13).

Comparable drugs:

Cetuximab (Erbitux).

Advantages:

• May be effective in some patients with colorectal cancer who have not responded to other therapies.

Disadvantages:

• Clinical benefit (e.g., prolonged survival) has not yet been demonstrated.
• Is not a first-line treatment for colorectal cancer.
• May be more likely to cause dermatologic toxicity.

Most important risks/adverse events:

Dermatologic toxicity (boxed warning; e.g., acneiform dermatitis, pruritus, erythema, rash, skin exfoliation, skin fissures, photosensitivity – patients should be advised to limit sun exposure and to wear sunscreen and a hat while undergoing treatment); severe infusion reactions (boxed warning; e.g., anaphylactic reaction, bronchospasm, fever, chills, hypotension); pulmonary fibrosis; hypomagnesemia (electrolyte concentrations should be periodically monitored during treatment and for 8 weeks following completion of therapy); diarrhea (when used in combination with irinotecan [Camptosar], may increase the incidence and severity of chemotherapy-induced diarrhea; combination use with an irinotecan/fluorouracil/leucovorin regimen is not recommended).

Most common adverse events:

Erythema (65%), acneiform dermatitis (57%), pruritus (57%), skin exfoliation (25%), paronychia (25%), rash (22%), skin fissures (20%), fatigue (26%), abdominal pain (25%), nausea (23%), diarrhea (21%), constipation (21%), hypomagnesemia (39%).

Usual dosage:

Identification of EGFR protein expression is necessary for the selection of patients for whom the use of the drug is appropriate; administered by intravenous infusion over a period of at least 60 minutes; 6 mg/kg administered over 60 minutes every 14 days; doses higher than 1,000 mg should be administered over 90 minutes.

Products:

Vials – 20 mg/mL, containing 5 mL (100 mg), 10 mL (200 mg), and 20 mL (400 mg); (should be stored in a refrigerator); volume of solution containing the needed dose should be diluted to a total of 100 mL with 0.9% Sodium Chloride Injection (doses higher than 1,000 mg should be diluted to 150 mL); should be administered via an intravenous infusion pump using a low-protein-binding 0.2 um or 0.22 um inline filter.

Comments:

Panitumumab is a human monoclonal antibody that, like cetuximab, binds to epidermal growth factor receptors (EGFR) and inhibits the growth and survival of selected human tumor cell lines expressing EGFR. In clinical studies, the mean progression-free survival in patients receiving panitumumab was 96 days compared with 60 days in those receiving best supportive care but not the new drug. Of the patients receiving panitumumab, 8% experienced a partial response whereas, in the control arm of the study, no patient had an objective response.

Pazopanib hydrochloride (Votrient – GlaxoSmithKline)
Antineoplastic Agent
2009

New Drug Comparison Rating (NDCR) = 3 (no or minor advantages/disadvantages)

Indication:
Treatment of patients with advanced renal cell carcinoma.

Comparable drugs:
Sorafenib (Nexavar), sunitinib (Sutent).

Advantages:
- May be less likely to cause left ventricular dysfunction.
- Less likely to cause hand-foot skin reaction (compared with sorafenib).
- Interacts with fewer medications (compared with sorafenib).
- Administered once a day (compared with sorafenib that is administered twice a day).

Disadvantages:
- Fewer labeled indications (sorafenib is also indicated for unresectable hepatocellular carcinoma and sunitinib is also indicated for gastrointestinal stromal tumor).
- Has not been directly compared with other antineoplastic agents in clinical studies.
- More likely to cause hepatotoxicity.
- Must be administered apart from food (compared with sunitinib that may be administered without regard to food).

Most important risks/adverse events:
Hepatotoxicity (boxed warning; serum transaminases [ALT, AST] and bilirubin should be determined before initiating treatment, at least once every 4 weeks for at least the first 4 months of treatment, and periodically thereafter; based on changes in liver function tests, treatment should be interrupted, reduced, or discontinued); QT interval prolongation (caution must be exercised in patients with risk factors); hemorrhagic events; arterial thrombotic events; gastrointestinal perforation and fistula; hypertension; hypothyroidism; proteinuria; impaired wound healing (treatment should be stopped at least 7 days prior to scheduled surgery); may cause harm to a fetus (Pregnancy Category D) and women of childbearing potential should avoid becoming pregnant while using the medication; use is not recommended in patients with severe hepatic impairment; is a substrate for CYP3A4 and action will be increased by strong CYP3A4 inhibitors (e.g., clarithromycin; concurrent use is best avoided; dosage reduction should be considered if used concurrently); action may be reduced by concurrent use of CYP3A4 inducers (e.g., carbamazepine; use of a medication with a lesser potential to interact should be considered); is a weak inhibitor of CYP3A4, CYP2C8, and CYP2D6, and concurrent use with substrates of these metabolic pathways is best avoided.

Most common adverse events:

Diarrhea (52%), hypertension (40%), hair color changes (38%), nausea (26%), anorexia (22%), vomiting (21%), fatigue (19%), ALT increased (53%), AST increased (53%), glucose increased (41%), total bilirubin increased (36%), leukopenia (37%), neutropenia (34%), thrombocytopenia (32%).

Usual dosage:

800 mg once a day at least 1 hour before or 2 hours after a meal; in patients with moderate hepatic impairment – 200 mg once a day; in patients also taking a strong CYP3A4 inhibitor – 400 mg once a day; systemic exposure and risk of adverse events are increased if drug is taken with food or if the tablets are crushed (tablets should not be crushed).

Products:

Tablets – 200 mg, 400 mg.

Comments:

Pazopanib is a multi-tyrosine kinase inhibitor of vascular endothelial growth factor (VEGF) receptors and has properties that are most similar to those of sunitinib and sorafenib. Other agents that have been recently approved for the treatment of advanced renal cell carcinoma include temsirolimus (Torisel), everolimus (Afinitor), and bevacizumab (Avastin). Pazopanib was evaluated in a placebo-controlled study in which progression-free survival averaged 9.2 months for patients receiving the drug compared to 4.2 months for those who did not receive the drug.

Pegaptanib sodium (Macugen — Eyetech; Pfizer)
Agent for Macular Degeneration
2005

New Drug Comparison Rating (NDCR) = 5 (important advance [see Comments])

Indication:
Administered by intravitreal injection for the treatment of neovascular (wet) age-related macular degeneration (AMD).

Comparable drugs:
Verteporfin (Visudyne); (subsequent to the marketing of pegaptanib, ranibizumab [Lucentis] has been marketed for the treatment of AMD).

Advantages:
- Labeled indication is more comprehensive (i.e., for treating all types of neovascular AMD).
- Unique mechanism of action for treating the disease (selective antagonism of vascular endothelial growth factor [VEGF] resulting in an antiangiogenesis action).
- Administration is less complex.

Disadvantages:
- Administered by intravitreous injection.
- Available only through a restricted distribution program.

Most important risks/adverse events:
Endophthalmitis (patients should be monitored [e.g., for reddening of the eye, sensitivity to light, change in vision] during the week following administration); contraindicated in patients with ocular or periocular infections.

Most common adverse events:
Ocular adverse events (incidence of 10% to 40%) including inflammation, blurred vision, cataracts, eye discharge, eye pain, visual disturbances, vitreous floaters, increased intraocular pressure (should be monitored).

Usual dosage:
0.3 mg via intravitreous injection every 6 weeks.

Product:
Syringes – 0.3 mg (should be stored in a refrigerator).

Comments:

Age-related macular degeneration (AMD) is a chronic, progressive disease of the macula that can result in the loss of central vision and blindness. In neovascular (wet) AMD, abnormal blood vessels leak blood and fluid into the retina resulting in damage to the macula and impairment of central vision. There are 3 subtypes of neovascular AMD—predominantly classic, minimally classic, and occult. Verteporfin was the first drug to be marketed (2000) for the treatment of AMD and it is specifically indicated for use in patients with the predominantly classic subtype. It is used in a 2-stage photodynamic treatment in which it is administered intravenously and then activated by shining nonthermal red laser light into the eye.

Vascular endothelial growth factor (VEGF) is a protein identified as a contributing factor in the occurrence of neovascular AMD. When VEGF is overexpressed, it promotes angiogenesis (blood vessel growth) and increased vascular permeability (leakage). Pegaptanib is a selective VEGF antagonist that targets the specific isoform VEGF 165 believed to be primarily responsible for the changes associated with ocular neovascularization. It is an aptamer (a single strand of nucleic acid that binds to a particular target) that represents a conjugate of an oligonucleotide of 28 nucleotides in length, terminating in a linker to which 2 monomethoxy polyethylene glycol units are covalently attached.

Pegaptanib has been approved for treating all neovascular AMD subtypes, providing an advantage over verteporfin. It does not restore vision in eyes damaged by AMD, but it can slow the rate of vision decline and help patients preserve the vision they have.

Although pegaptanib represented an important advance when it was marketed in 2005, its importance has decreased with the subsequent marketing of ranibizumab in 2006.

Plerixafor (Mozobil – Genzyme)
Hematopoietic stem cell mobilizer
2009

New Drug Comparison Rating (NDCR) = 4 (significant advantages)

Indication:

Administered subcutaneously for use in combination with granulocyte-colony stimulating factor (G-CSF) to mobilize hematopoietic stem cells to the peripheral blood for collection and subsequent autologous transplantation in patients with non-Hodgkin's lymphoma and multiple myeloma.

Comparable drugs:

Granulocyte-colony stimulating factor (G-CSF; filgrastim [Neupogen]), granulocyte-macrophage colony stimulating factor (sargramostim [Leukine]).

Advantages:

- Unique mechanism of action (inhibits stem cell CXCR4 that has a role in anchoring these cells to the marrow matrix).
- Significantly increases the number of stem cells collected from the peripheral blood.

Disadvantages:

- Has not been evaluated for use as a single agent.

Most important risks/adverse events:

Should not be used in patients with leukemia because leukemic cells may be mobilized; potential for release of tumor cells from marrow; hematologic effects (increased circulating leukocytes, decreased platelets [blood cell counts and platelet counts should be monitored]); potential for splenic rupture; may cause harm to a fetus (Pregnancy Category D) and women of childbearing potential should be advised to not become pregnant during the period of use of the drug.

Most common adverse events:

Diarrhea (37%), nausea (34%), injection site reactions (34%), dizziness (11%), vomiting (10%).

Usual dosage:

Administered subcutaneously; patients should first receive daily morning doses of G-CSF (10 mcg/kg) for 4 days prior to the first evening dose of plerixafor and on each day prior to apheresis; plerixafor is administered in the evening approximately 11 hours before initiating apheresis for up to 4 consecutive days; recommended dosage is 0.24 mg/kg body weight; dosage is calculated based on actual body weight in patients up to 175% of ideal body weight; dosage should not exceed 40 mg a day; in patients with moderate and severe renal impairment (creatinine clearance less than or equal to 50 mL/minute), the dosage should be reduced to 0.16 mg per kg once a day, with a maximum dosage of 27 mg once a day.

Product:

Single-use vials – containing 1.2 mL of a solution of the drug in a 20 mg/mL concentration.

Comments:

The use of bone marrow transplants in the treatment of certain blood cancers such as multiple myeloma and non-Hodgkin's lymphomas has permitted the use of dosages of chemotherapy and radiotherapy that are higher than those that would ordinarily be considered safe to use. Hematopoietic stem cells mature into blood cells such as red blood cells, white blood cells, and platelets. These stem cells are primarily located in the bone marrow. Stem cells that leave the bone marrow and circulate into the blood are called peripheral blood stem cells (PBSCs). However, usually few PBSCs exist in the blood because of the extent to which the stem cells bind to, or are anchored by, the bone marrow. G-CSF (filgrastim) and sargramostim have been used to mobilize the transfer of hematopoietic stem cells from the bone marrow to the peripheral blood. Plerixafor is indicated for use in combination with G-CSF. By inhibiting CXCR4 chemokine receptors, it facilitates the release of stem cells that are anchored to the marrow matrix, resulting in more stem cells being transferred to peripheral blood for collection during apheresis. In a study in patients with non-Hodgkin's lymphoma, 59% of the patients receiving plerixafor and G-CSF collected approximately the same number of stem cells from the peripheral blood in four or fewer apheresis sessions as 20% of the patients receiving placebo and G-CSF. In a study in patients with multiple myeloma, 72% of the patients receiving plerixafor and G-CSF collected approximately the same number of stem cells in two or fewer apheresis sessions as 34% of the patients receiving placebo and G-CSF.

Posaconazole (Noxafil – Schering)
Antifungal Agent
2006

New Drug Comparison Rating (NDCR) = 4 (significant advantages)

Indications:

Prophylaxis of invasive Aspergillus and Candida infections in patients 13 years of age and older who are at high risk of developing these infections due to being severely immunocompromised, such as hematopoietic stem cell transplant (HSCT) recipients with graft-versus-host disease (GVHD) or those with hematologic malignancies who develop prolonged neutropenia from chemotherapy; treatment of oropharyngeal candidiasis including oropharyngeal candidiasis refractory to itraconazole and/or fluconazole.

Comparable drugs:

Fluconazole (e.g., Diflucan), itraconazole (e.g., Sporanox), voriconazole (Vfend).

Advantages:

- First drug approved for prophylaxis against invasive Aspergillus infection.
- More effective in preventing invasive Aspergillus infection.
- May be effective in oropharyngeal candidiasis that is refractory to other agents.
- Less likely to cause visual disturbances (compared with voriconazole).

Disadvantages:

- Fewer labeled indications.
- Absorption and activity may be less predictable.
- Not available in a parenterally-administered formulation.

Most important risks/adverse events:

Hepatic adverse events (liver function tests should be monitored); inhibits the CYP3A4 metabolic pathway and concurrent use with sirolimus (Rapamune) or ergot-type products is contraindicated (concurrent use with other CYP3A4 substrates [e.g., cyclosporine (e.g., Neoral), tacrolimus (Prograf)] should be closely monitored; QT interval prolongation (concurrent use with other drugs that prolong the QT interval and are metabolized via the CYP3A4 pathway [e.g., quinidine, pimozide (e.g., Orap)] is contraindicated); may increase the action of digoxin; action may be reduced by cimetidine (e.g., Tagamet), efavirenz (Sustiva), phenytoin (e.g., Dilantin), and rifabutin (e.g., Mycobutin), and concurrent use is best avoided.

Most common adverse events:

Nausea (7%), vomiting (5%), diarrhea (5%).

Usual dosage:

Should be administered with a full meal or with a liquid nutritional supplement if the patient cannot eat a full meal; prophylaxis – 200 mg 3 times a day; treatment (oropharyngeal candidiasis) – 100 mg twice a day on the first day, then 100 mg once a day for 13 days; oropharyngeal candidiasis that is refractory to itraconazole and/or fluconazole – 400 mg twice a day; in patients taking cyclosporine or tacrolimus, the dosage of the immunosuppressant should be reduced.

Product:

Oral suspension – 40 mg/mL.

Comments:

Posaconazole is a triazole antifungal agent with properties that are most similar to those of fluconazole and itraconazole. It is effective in preventing certain invasive fungal infections in patients who are at high risk of serious consequences from such infections, and is the first drug to be approved for prophylaxis against invasive Aspergillus infection. When compared with fluconazole and itraconazole, substantially fewer breakthrough infections caused by Aspergillus species occurred in patients receiving prophylaxis with posaconazole.

Although posaconazole is not a substrate for CYP3A4, it does inhibit this metabolic pathway and may increase the action of numerous other medications that are substrates. Posaconazole is incompletely absorbed following oral administration, but its bioavailability and peak concentrations are 3 to 4 times higher when it is administered with a meal relative to a fasting state. Therefore, it should be administered with a full meal or a liquid nutritional supplement.

Pralatrexate (Folotyn – Allos)
Antineoplastic Agent
2009

New Drug Comparison Rating (NDCR) = 4 (significant advantages)

Indication:

Administered intravenously for the treatment of patients with relapsed or refractory peripheral T-cell lymphoma (PTCL).

Comparable drug:

Methotrexate.

Advantages:

- Is the first drug to be approved for the treatment of PTCL.

Disadvantages:

- Has not been approved as a first-line treatment of PTCL.
- Has not been directly compared with other antineoplastic agents in clinical studies.
- Must be administered intravenously.

Most important risks/adverse events:

Bone marrow suppression (thrombocytopenia, neutropenia, anemia; dosage modifications are based on ANC and platelet count prior to each dose); mucositis (if severity is grade 2 or greater, dosage should be modified); to potentially reduce treatment-related hematological toxicity and mucositis, supplementation with folic acid (1 – 1.25 mg daily starting during the 10-day period prior to the first dose and continuing for 30 days following the last dose) and vitamin B12 (1 mg intramuscularly no more than 10 weeks prior to the first dose and every 8-10 weeks thereafter) should be provided; complete blood cell counts and severity of mucositis should be monitored weekly; serum chemistry tests, including renal and hepatic function, should be performed prior to the start of the first and fourth dose of a given cycle; may cause harm to a fetus (Pregnancy Category D) and women of childbearing potential should be advised to avoid becoming pregnant; renal clearance may be delayed by concurrent administration of probenecid, trimethoprim/sulfamethoxazole, or nonsteroidal anti-inflammatory drugs.

Most common adverse events:

Mucositis (70%), thrombocytopenia (41%), nausea (40%), fatigue (36%), anemia (34%), constipation (33%), pyrexia (32%), edema (30%), cough (28%), epistaxis (26%), vomiting (25%), neutropenia (24%).

153

Usual dosage:

30 mg/m^2 administered as an intravenous push over 3 - 5 minutes via the side port of a free flowing 0.9% Sodium Chloride Injection intravenous line once weekly for 6 weeks in 7-week cycles until progressive disease or unacceptable toxicity; product labeling should be consulted for dosage modifications based on hematologic toxicities, mucositis, and liver function test abnormalities.

Product:

Single-use vials – 20 mg/mL (vials contain 1 mL or 2 mL of solution); should be stored in a refrigerator; solution does not require dilution prior to administration.

Comments:

Peripheral T-cell lymphoma (PTCL) is one of the non-Hodgkin's lymphomas and occurs in less than 10,000 patients each year in the United States. Most patients have been treated with cyclophosphamide, doxorubicin, vincristine, and prednisone, or a similar regimen, but none of these agents has been specifically approved for the treatment of PTCL. Many patients are refractory to these regimens or experience relapses. Pralatrexate is a folate analog metabolic inhibitor that has properties that are most similar to those of methotrexate. It competitively inhibits dihydrofolate reductase and is the first drug to be approved for the treatment of PTCL, although its specific indication is for the treatment of patients with relapsed or refractory PTCL rather than first-line use. In the clinical study in which it was evaluated in patients with relapsed or refractory PTCL, the response rate was 27% with approximately two-thirds of these patients experiencing a partial response.

Pramlintide acetate (Symlin – Amylin)
Antidiabetic Agent
2005

New Drug Comparison Rating (NDCR) = 4 (significant advantages)

Indications:

Administered subcutaneously in patients with type 1 and type 2 diabetes mellitus as an adjunct treatment in patients who use mealtime insulin therapy and who have failed to achieved desired glycemic control despite optimal insulin therapy; use in conjunction with mealtime insulin therapy in patients with type 2 diabetes may be with or without concurrent metformin and/or sulfonylurea therapy.

Comparable drugs:

Insulin.

Advantages:

- Has a unique mechanism of action (acts as an amylinomimetic agent).
- May improve glycemic control in patients for whom optimal insulin therapy has not provided the desired control.
- Use may result in weight loss.

Disadvantages:

- Increases the risk of insulin-induced hypoglycemia.
- Causes nausea in many patients.
- May reduce the absorption and activity of certain orally administered drugs.
- Cannot be mixed with insulin.

Most important risks/adverse events:

Hypoglycemia, particularly in patients with type 1 diabetes (boxed warning); slows gastric emptying and is contraindicated in patients with gastroparesis; should not be used in patients who are taking drugs that alter gastrointestinal motility (e.g., anticholinergic agents) or slow the absorption of nutrients (e.g., alpha-glucosidase inhibitors [e.g., miglitol]); medications such as analgesics, for which a rapid onset of action is important, should be administered at least 1 hour before or 2 hours after pramlintide.

Most common adverse events (incidences in patients with type 1 and type 2 diabetes, respectively):

Nausea (48%, 28%), anorexia (17%, 9%), vomiting (11%, 8%), fatigue (7%, 7%), inflicted injury (14%, less than 5%), headache (less than 5%, 13%).

Usual dosage:

Administered subcutaneously immediately prior to major meals; when initiating therapy, the dosage of preprandial, rapid-acting or short-acting insulins should be reduced by 50%; type 1 diabetes – initiate treatment at a dose of 15 mcg and titrate at 15 mcg increments to a maintenance dose of 30 mcg or 60 mcg as tolerated; type 2 diabetes – initial dosage of 60 mcg immediately prior to major meals, with a subsequent increase in the dose to 120 mcg.

Products:

Vials – 0.6 mg/mL (should be stored in a refrigerator).

Comments:

Amylin is secreted with insulin by pancreatic beta cells in response to food intake. In patients with diabetes who need insulin, these pancreatic cells are dysfunctional or damaged and both insulin and amylin secretion in response to food is reduced. Pramlintide is a synthetic analogue of human amylin and acts as an amylinomimetic agent. It affects the rate of postprandial glucose appearance by several mechanisms including slowing gastric emptying, suppressing glucagon secretion, and reducing total caloric intake.

Although pramlintide itself does not cause hypoglycemia, it is used with insulin therapy and increases the risk of insulin-induced severe hypoglycemia, particularly in patients with type 1 diabetes. The risk of severe hypoglycemia is greatest during the first 3 hours following pramlintide injection and could result in injury if patients are engaged in high-risk activities during that period of time. Accordingly, caution must be exercised in selecting patients for treatment, frequent pre- and post-meal glucose monitoring should be performed, and there should be an initial 50% reduction in the pre-meal insulin doses.

Prasugrel hydrochloride (Effient – Daiichi Sankyo; Lilly)
Antiplatelet Agent
2009

New Drug Comparison Rating (NDCR) = 4 (significant advantages)

Indication:

To reduce the rate of thrombotic cardiovascular events (including stent thrombosis) in patients with acute coronary syndrome (ACS) who are to be managed with percutaneous coronary intervention (PCI), including patients with unstable angina or non-ST-elevation myocardial infarction (NSTEMI), and patients with ST-elevation myocardial infarction (STEMI) when managed with primary or delayed PCI.

Comparable drugs:

Clopidogrel (Plavix).

Advantages:

- Is more effective in reducing nonfatal myocardial infarction and stent thrombosis.
- Action is not likely to be changed by genetic influences that reduce CYP2C19 activity.
- Action is not likely to be reduced by the concurrent use of CYP2C19 inhibitors (e.g., omeprazole).
- May be less likely to cause thrombotic thrombocytopenic purpura.

Disadvantages:

- Is more likely to cause bleeding (boxed warning).
- Is contraindicated in patients with a history of prior transient ischemic attack (TIA) or stroke.
- Labeled indications are more limited (indications for clopidogrel also include use in patients with NSTEMI who are to be managed medically or with coronary artery bypass graft (CABG) surgery, and for the reduction of atherothrombotic events in patients with a history of recent myocardial infarction, recent stroke, or established peripheral arterial disease).
- Use should generally be avoided in patients 75 years of age and older because of an increased risk of bleeding (except in high-risk situations such as in patients with diabetes).

Most important risks/adverse events:

Contraindicated in patients with active pathological bleeding (e.g., peptic ulcer, intracranial hemorrhage), and in patients with a history of prior (TIA) or stroke; bleeding risk (boxed warning) with risk factors for bleeding including bodyweight less than 60 kg, propensity to bleed (e.g., recent trauma), concomitant use of medications that increase the risk of bleeding (e.g., warfarin, heparin, chronic use of nonsteroidal anti-inflammatory drugs), and age of 75 years and older; treatment should not be started in patients likely to undergo urgent CABG surgery; where possible, treatment should be discontinued at least 7 days prior to any surgery; if bleeding occurs, efforts should be made to manage it without discontinuing treatment as this may increase the risk of subsequent cardiovascular events.

Most common adverse events:

Non-CABG-related major or minor bleeding (5%), hypertension (8%), hypercholesterolemia/hyperlipidemia (7%), headache (6%), back pain (5%), dyspnea (5%), nausea (5%).

Usual dosage:

A single loading dose of 60 mg, followed with a maintenance dosage of 10 mg once a day; patients should also be treated with aspirin in a dosage of 75 mg to 325 mg daily; in patients weighing less than 60 kg, decreasing the maintenance dosage to 5 mg once a day should be considered.

Products:

Tablets – 5 mg, 10 mg.

Comments:

Prasugrel is a thienopyridine derivative that is structurally and pharmacologically related to clopidogrel and ticlopidine (e.g., Ticlid). Like these other agents, prasugrel is a prodrug that is converted to an active metabolite that inhibits platelet activation and aggregation by binding to the P2Y12 class of adenosine 5' diphosphate (ADP) receptors on platelets. Whereas the conversion of clopidogrel to its active metabolite primarily involves the CYP2C19 pathway, the involvement of this pathway in the conversion of prasugrel to its active metabolite is limited, and the action of prasugrel is not likely to be influenced by genetic variations in CYP2C19 activity or the concurrent use of a CYP2C19 inhibitor such as omeprazole.

The effectiveness of prasugrel was demonstrated in studies in which it was used in conjunction with aspirin and compared with a regimen of clopidogrel and aspirin. The prasugrel/aspirin regimen provided a 19% relative risk reduction with the greater effectiveness almost entirely attributable to a reduction in nonfatal myocardial infarction. There were also fewer stent-related clots (i.e., stent thrombosis) in patients treated with prasugrel/aspirin, with a relative risk reduction of approximately 50%. The greater effectiveness of prasugrel in the treatment of patients with ACS who are to be managed with PCI should be considered in the context of a greater risk of bleeding that necessitates stronger warnings and restrictions for the new drug, as well as much more limited labeled indications when compared with clopidogrel.

Opinions differ regarding the results of the clinical studies and some have proposed that, if a lower dosage of prasugrel had been used, there might be little or no difference in the efficacy of prasugrel and clopidogrel, as well as the risk of bleeding. The labeling for prasugrel also includes an "alternative explanation" for the differences reported in the comparison of the two drugs, that being the lack of an evaluation of the possibility that the action of clopidogrel may have been reduced in some patients because of genetic influences that reduced the activity of the CYP2C19 metabolic pathway, or the concurrent use of a CYP2C19 inhibitor such as omeprazole.

Pregabalin (Lyrica – Pfizer)
Agent for Neuropathic Pain
2005

New Drug Comparison Rating (NDCR) = 3 (no or minor advantages/disadvantages [see Comments])

Indications:

Management of neuropathic pain associated with diabetic peripheral neuropathy; management of postherpetic neuralgia; adjunctive therapy for adult patients with partial onset seizures; (subsequently approved for the management of fibromyalgia).

Comparable drugs:

Gabapentin (e.g., Neurontin).

Advantages:

- Has a labeled indication for neuropathic pain associated with diabetic peripheral neuropathy.
- May be administered 2 (or 3) times a day for the treatment of postherpetic neuralgia and partial onset seizures (compared to 3 times a day with gabapentin).
- Attainment of optimum dosage may be easier.

Disadvantages:

- Is a controlled substance (Schedule V).
- May be more likely to cause musculoskeletal adverse events and CK elevations.
- May reduce platelet counts.
- Has not been evaluated in pediatric patients.

Most important risks/adverse events:

Dizziness and somnolence (patients should be cautioned about engaging in potentially hazardous activities); musculoskeletal effects/creatine kinase (CK) elevations (patients should promptly report unexplained muscle pain, tenderness, or weakness); withdrawal symptoms (is a controlled substance in Schedule V); decreased platelet count; tumorigenic potential (based on studies in mice); male-mediated teratogenicity (based on studies in rats)(labeling has been subsequently revised to include a warning about suicidal thinking and behavior).

Most common adverse events:

Dizziness (26%), somnolence (16%), peripheral edema (12%), dry mouth (8%), headache (7%), infection (7%), ataxia (5%), blurred vision (5%), constipation (5%), euphoria (4%), abnormal gait (4%), weight gain (4%).

Usual dosage:

Neuropathic pain associated with diabetic peripheral neuropathy – 50 mg 3 times a day initially and increased to 100 mg 3 times a day within 1 week; postherpetic neuralgia – 75 mg 2 times a day or 50 mg 3 times a day initially and increased to 300 mg a day (divided into 2 or 3 doses) within 1 week; partial onset seizures – 75 mg 2 times a day or 50 mg 3 times a day initially and increased to a maximum of 600 mg a day divided into 2 or 3 doses; fibromyalgia – 75 mg two times a day initially and increased to 150 mg two times a day within 1 week and subsequently to 225 mg two times a day; dosage increases are based on an assessment of efficacy and tolerability; dosage should be reduced in patients with renal impairment; when treatment is to be discontinued, dosage should be reduced gradually over a minimum of 1 week.

Products:

Capsules – 25 mg, 50 mg, 75 mg, 100 mg, 150 mg, 200 mg, 225 mg, 300 mg.

Comments:

Pregabalin is structurally related to gabapentin and has many properties similar to those of the older drug. Their mechanism(s) of action may involve modulation of calcium channel function resulting in the reduction of calcium-dependent release of several neurotransmitters. Pregabalin is the first prescription medication to be approved for the management of neuropathic pain associated with both postherpetic neuralgia and diabetic peripheral neuropathy. Although gabapentin is widely used for neuropathic pain associated with diabetic peripheral neuropathy, it is not a labeled indication.

Titration of the dosage of pregabalin to obtain the optimum balance of benefit and risk is more easily accomplished than with the use of gabapentin. Pregabalin is primarily excreted in the urine in unchanged form and its dosage should be reduced in patients with renal impairment.

The NDCR of 3 for pregabalin was based, in part, on the indications for which it was initially approved that did not include fibromyalgia, for which it was approved in 2007.

Raltegravir (Isentress – Merck)
Antiviral Agent
2007

New Drug Comparison Rating (NDCR) = 4 (significant advantages)

Indication:

In combination with other antiretroviral agents for the treatment of HIV-1 infection in treatment-experienced adult patients who have evidence of viral replication and HIV-1 strains resistant to multiple antiretroviral agents (has been subequently revised to delete "tretment-experienced" and "who have evidence of viral replication and HIV-1 strains resistant to multiple antiretroviral agents").

Comparable drugs:

Other antiretroviral agents; comparisons are made with the HIV protease inhibitors (e.g., lopinavir/ritonavir [Kaletra], atazanavir [Reyataz], darunavir [Prezista]).

Advantages:

- Has a unique mechanism of action (inhibits HIV integrase strand transfer).
- Is effective in some patients who have become resistant to other regimens.
- Use is associated with fewer serious adverse events.
- Interacts with fewer medications.

Disadvantages:

- Use is limited to treatment-experienced patients with evidence of resistance to other agents (except for darunavir and tipranavir [Aptivus], as well as enfuvirtide [Fuzeon] and maraviroc [Selzentry], whose use is also limited to treatment-experienced patients).
- May be more likely to increase creatine kinase (CK) concentrations and cause musculoskeletal adverse events.
- Is administered twice a day (compared with atazanavir that is administered once a day).

Most important risks/adverse events:

Immune reconstitution syndrome; is primarily eliminated by metabolism via a uridine diphosphate glucuronosyltransferase (UGT) 1A1-mediated glucuronidation pathway and action may be reduced by the concurrent use of a strong inducer of UGT1A1 such as rifampin (e.g., Rifadin); may increase creatine kinase (CK) concentrations – myopathy and rhabdomyolysis have been reported and caution should be exercised in patients who are also being treated with other medications (e.g., statins [e.g., atorvastatin (Lipitor)]) that are known to cause these conditions; (rash and severe skin reactions have been reported in the postmarketing experience).

Most common adverse events:

Diarrhea (17%), nausea (10%), headache (10%), pyrexia (5%).

Usual dosage:

400 mg twice a day (subsequently revised to include a dosage recommendation of 800 mg twice a day in patients also being treated with rifampin).

Product:

Tablets – 400 mg.

Comments:

Like HIV protease and reverse transcriptase, integrase is an HIV-1 enzyme that has an important role in the replication of the virus by facilitating the integration of viral DNA into the DNA of host cells. Raltegravir has a unique mechanism of action and is designated as an HIV integrase strand transfer inhibitor (integrase inhibitor). The inhibition of integration by raltegravir blocks propagation of the viral infection. Additive to synergistic antiretroviral activity has been demonstrated in cell cultures when raltegravir has been combined with most other antiretroviral agents.

Raltegravir joins darunavir, tipranavir, enfuvirtide, and maraviroc as antiretroviral agents that are not indicated for inclusion in initial regimens for the treatment of HIV infection, but are of value when reserved for use in patients who demonstrate resistance to previous regimens. The effectiveness of raltegravir in reducing HIV-1 RNA concentrations was demonstrated in two controlled studies in patients with documented resistance to at least one drug in each of three classes of antiretroviral agents. Patients received either raltegravir or placebo in addition to optimized background therapy (OBT) consisting of two to seven antiretroviral agents.

Although experience with raltegravir is limited, it appears less likely than most other antiretroviral agents to cause serious adverse events or to interact with other medications. The discontinuation rate (2%) in the clinical studies due to adverse events was similar to that in the group receiving placebo plus OBT.

Ramelteon (Rozerem – Takeda)
Hypnotic
2005

New Drug Comparison Rating (NDCR) = 4 (significant advantages)

Indication:
Treatment of insomnia characterized by difficulty with sleep onset.

Comparable drugs:
Eszopiclone (Lunesta), zaleplon (Sonata), zolpidem (Ambien), temazepam (e.g., Restoril).

Advantages:
- Unique mechanism of action (melatonin receptor agonist).
- Not associated with a risk of dependence and is not a controlled substance.
- Short duration of action and is not likely to cause daytime sedation (compared with eszopiclone, zolpidem, and temazepam).

Disadvantages:
- Less effective in improving sleep maintenance because of short duration of action (compared with eszopiclone, zolpidem, and temazepam).
- Action is increased by the concurrent use of a strong CYP1A2 inhibitor (e.g., fluvoxamine).
- Pregnancy Category C (compared with zolpidem, which is Category B).
- Long-term use may increase prolactin concentrations and decrease testosterone concentrations.

Most important risks/adverse events:
Is extensively metabolized via the CYP1A2 pathway and should not be used concurrently with fluvoxamine (e.g., Luvox), a potent CYP1A2 inhibitor; concurrent use with a potent CYP3A4 inhibitor (e.g., clarithromycin [e.g., Biaxin]) should be closely monitored; should not be used in patients with severe hepatic impairment; has not been studied in patients with severe sleep apnea or severe chronic obstructive pulmonary disease and its use is not recommended in patients with these disorders.

Most common adverse events:
Somnolence (5%), dizziness (5%), fatigue (4%).

Usual dosage:
8 mg taken within 30 minutes of going to bed; should not be administered with or immediately after a high-fat meal.

Product:

Tablets – 8 mg.

Comments:

The natural hormone melatonin has been thought to help regulate the sleep-wake cycle by stimulating melatonin receptors in the suprachiasmatic nucleus in the brain, and dietary supplements containing melatonin have been widely used for insomnia and by travelers adjusting to different time zones. However, studies demonstrating the effectiveness of these products have been very limited.

Ramelteon is structurally related to melatonin and is a melatonin receptor agonist with a high affinity for melatonin MT1 and MT2 receptors that are considered to be involved in the maintenance of the circadian rhythm underlying the normal sleep-wake cycle. Melatonin also has a high affinity for MT3 receptors, but the influence of this receptor type on the sleep-wake cycle is not as well understood.

Ramelteon is the first drug approved for insomnia that acts via a mechanism other than a central nervous system depressant action. Unlike the other hypnotics available on prescription, its use does not appear to be associated with a risk of dependence and it is not classified as a controlled substance. It is effective in the treatment of insomnia characterized by difficulty with sleep onset (i.e., falling asleep). Because it has a shorter duration of action than most of the other hypnotics (zaleplon being an exception), it is likely to be less effective in insomnia characterized by difficulty maintaining sleep. However, its short duration of action is an advantage with respect to a lesser likelihood of daytime sedation.

Ranibizumab (Lucentis – Genentech)
Agent for Macular Degeneration
2006

New Drug Comparison Rating (NDCR) = 5 (important advance)

Indication:
Administered by intravitreal injection for the treatment of patients with neovascular (wet) age-related macular degeneration (AMD).

Comparable drugs:
Pegaptanib (Macugen), verteporfin (Visudyne).

Advantages:
- First drug to provide improvement in vision.
- Maintains vision after 12 and 24 months.
- Indicated for treatment of all subtypes of neovascular AMD (compared with verteporfin).

Disadvantages:
- Administered by intravitreous injection (compared with verteporfin).

Most important risks/adverse events:
Contraindicated in patients with ocular or periocular infections; endophthalmitis; retinal detachment; patients should be monitored during the week following each injection.

Most common adverse events (probably often attributable to the injection procedure rather than to the medication):
Conjunctival hemorrhage (60%), eye pain (27%), vitreous floaters (27%), retinal hemorrhage (21%).

Usual dosage:
0.5 mg (0.05 mL) via intravitreal injection once a month; frequency of administration may be reduced to once every 3 months after the first 4 injections, if monthly injections are not feasible (however, this modified regimen is less effective than the monthly regimen).

Product:
Vials – 0.5 mg in 0.05 mL (should be stored in a refrigerator).

Comments:

Ranibizumab is a recombinant humanized immunoglobulin G1 kappa isotype monoclonal antibody fragment that binds to vascular endothelial growth factor-A (VEGF-A) and prevents its interaction with its receptors. In one of the clinical studies, 95% of patients maintained their vision after 12 months, and 90% after 24 months. Approximately one-third of the patients experienced improved vision after 12 and 24 months, and it is the first drug demonstrated to be effective in improving vision in a substantial percentage of patients. In another study, it was compared with verteporfin PDT (photodynamic therapy) and, after 12 months, 96% of patients treated with ranibizumab maintained their vision and 40% experienced improved vision, compared with 64% and 6%, respectively, in those receiving verteporfin PDT. Ranibizumab has not been directly compared with pegaptanib but the results of the separate studies of the two agents suggest that the latter agent is less effective. The antineoplastic agent, bevacizumab (Avastin), is related to ranibizumab and is also a VEGF inhibitor. It has been used "off-label" in the treatment of AMD but has not been directly compared with ranibizumab.

Ranolazine (Ranexa – Gilead)
Antianginal Agent
2006

New Drug Comparison Rating (NDCR) = 4 (significant advantages)

Indication:

Treatment of chronic angina; should be reserved for patients who have not achieved an adequate response with other antianginal drugs; should be used in combination with amlodipine (Norvasc), a beta-blocker, or nitrate; (subsequently revised to remove limitation of reserving its use for patients who have not achieved an adequate response with other agents; labeling now notes that it may be used with beta-blockers, nitrates, calcium channel blockers, anti-platelet therapy, lipid-lowering therapy, ACE inhibitors, and angiotensin receptor blockers).

Comparable drugs:

Amlodipine (Norvasc), beta-blockers (e.g., atenolol [e.g., Tenormin]), long-acting nitrates (e.g., isosorbide mononitrate [e.g., Imdur]).

Advantages:

- Unique mechanism of action.
- May increase the effectiveness of antianginal regimens in some patients in whom the previous regimens did not provide an adequate response.

Disadvantages:

- May cause QT interval prolongation.
- Interacts with more medications.
- Contraindicated in patients with hepatic impairment.

Most important risks/adverse events:

Contraindicated in patients with clinically significant hepatic impairment; concurrent use with a strong CYP3A inhibitor (e.g., clarithromycin [e.g., Biaxin]) or a CYP3A inducer (e.g., rifampin [e.g., Rifadin]) is contraindicated; action may be increased by the concurrent use of a moderate CYP3A inhibitor (e.g., diltiazem [e.g., Cardizem], verapamil [e.g., Covera-HS]); may cause QT prolongation and caution must be exercised in patients who are taking other QT-prolonging drugs (e.g., antiarrhythmic agents); may increase the action of digoxin.

Most common adverse events:

Dizziness (6%), headache (6%), constipation (5%), nausea (4%).

Usual dosage:

500 mg twice a day; may be increased to 1000 mg twice a day; dosage should not exceed 500 mg twice a day in patients who are also taking a moderate CYP3A inhibitor (e.g., diltiazem, verapamil) concurrently.

Product:

Extended-release tablets – 500 mg, 1000 mg.

Comments:

Ranolazine is a late sodium current inhibitor but the specific mechanisms through which it provides its antianginal and anti-ischemic effects have not been identified. However, the clinical benefit attributed to its use does not depend on reductions in heart rate or blood pressure. Ranolazine prolongs the QT interval in a dose-related manner. Although problems associated with this effect were not identified in the clinical studies, other drugs causing this response have been associated with the occurrence of serious arrhythmias. When it was initially approved, the labeled indication for ranolazine limited its use to patients with chronic angina that had not responded adequately to other antianginal regimens. However, in late 2008, the labeling was revised to remove this limitation. When ranolazine is to be used in conjunction with a calcium channel blocking agent, amlodipine is often the best choice; concurrent use with diltiazem or verapamil may increase the action of ranolazine.

In addition to being a substrate for CYP3A, ranolazine is a substrate for P-glycoprotein (P-gp) and caution should be exercised when it is used concurrently with a P-gp inhibitor such as cyclosporine (e.g., Neoral). Ranolazine may inhibit the CYP3A, CYP2D6, and P-gp metabolic pathways. It has been reported to increase the concentrations of digoxin, a P-gp substrate, and simvastatin (e.g., Zocor), a CYP3A substrate.

Rasagiline mesylate (Azilect – Teva Neuroscience)
Antiparkinson Agent
2006

New Drug Comparison Rating (NDCR) = 3 (no or minor advantages/disadvantages)

Indication:
Treatment of the signs and symptoms of idiopathic Parkinson's disease as initial monotherapy and as adjunct therapy to levodopa.

Comparable drugs:
Selegiline (e.g., Eldepryl, Zelapar).

Advantages:
- Labeled indications include initial monotherapy.
- Is administered once a day (compared with Eldepryl and generic formulations that are administered twice a day; however, Zelapar is administered once a day).
- Is not converted to amphetamine metabolites.

Disadvantages:
- Consumption of tyramine-rich foods, beverages, and dietary supplements should be restricted.
- Labeling is more restrictive with respect to the potential for interactions with other drugs (e.g., concurrent use with a larger number of drugs is contraindicated).
- Interacts with CYP1A2 inhibitors (e.g., ciprofloxacin, fluvoxamine).

Most important risks/adverse events:
Because of its monoamine oxidase (MAO) inhibitory action, concurrent use is contraindicated with cyclobenzaprine (e.g., Flexeril), dextromethorphan, meperidine (e.g., Demerol), methadone, mirtazapine (Remeron), other MAO inhibitors (e.g., selegiline [e.g., Eldepryl], tranylcypromine [e.g., Parnate]), propoxyphene (e.g., Darvon), St. John's wort, sympathomimetic amines (e.g., amphetamines, phenylephrine, pseudoephedrine), and tramadol (e.g., Ultram); concurrent use with a tricyclic antidepressant (e.g., amitriptyline), selective serotonin reuptake inhibitor (e.g., fluoxetine [e.g., Prozac]), or serotonin-norepinephrine reuptake inhibitor (e.g., venlafaxine [Effexor]) is best avoided; consumption of tyramine-rich foods (e.g., aged cheeses), beverages (e.g., red wines), or dietary supplements should be restricted; is extensively metabolized (primarily via the CYP1A2 pathway) and action may be increased by the concurrent use of a CYP1A2 inhibitor (e.g., ciprofloxacin [e.g., Cipro], fluvoxamine [e.g., Luvox]); should not be used in patients with moderate or severe hepatic impairment (labeling has subsequently been revised to reduce medication and food restrictions).

Most common adverse events:

Arthralgia (7%), dyspepsia (7%), depression (5%), flu syndrome (5%), fall (5%); potential for postural hypotension is greater in patients treated with rasagiline and levodopa.

Usual dosage:

As monotherapy, 1 mg once a day; as an adjunct to levodopa, 0.5 mg once a day initially, with a subsequent increase to 1 mg once a day, if needed; dosage of 0.5 mg once a day should be used in patients with mild hepatic impairment or in patients treated with a CYP1A2 inhibitor.

Products:

Tablets – 0.5 mg, 1 mg.

Comments:

Rasagiline is a selective inhibitor of monoamine oxidase type B (MAO-B) and has properties that are most similar to those of selegiline. Their inhibition of MAO-B results in increased dopamine concentrations in the striatum. Both agents are indicated as adjunct therapy to levodopa, and rasagiline is also indicated as initial monotherapy. However, neither agent is likely to be used often as initial monotherapy.

Rasagiline and selegiline probably have a similar risk for adverse events and drug interactions related to their MAO inhibitory activity when used in the recommended dosages. However, a dosage has been identified for selegiline that is not likely to be associated with a risk of interactions with tyramine-containing dietary items, but such a dosage has hot yet been established for rasagiline. Accordingly, there are prominent warnings in the labeling for rasagiline, but not selegiline, about the need to restrict dietary tyramine. In addition, the labeling for rasagiline identifies a larger number of drugs with which concurrent use is contraindicated.

Retapamulin (Altabax — GlaxoSmithKline)
Antibacterial Agent
2007

New Drug Comparison Rating (NDCR) = 4 (significant advantages)

Indication:

For topical application in adults and pediatric patients aged 9 months and older for the treatment of impetigo (up to 100 cm^2 in total area in adults or 2% total body surface area in pediatric patients aged 9 months or older) caused by Staphylococcus aureus (methicillin-susceptible isolates only) or Streptococcus pyogenes.

Comparable drug:

Mupirocin (e.g., Bactroban).

Advantages:

- Less frequent administration (twice a day compared with three times a day).
- Shorter course of treatment (five days compared with at least eight days).
- First of a new class of antibacterial agents (pleuromutilins).
- Unique mechanism of action, and cross-resistance with other antibacterial agents has not been reported.

Disadvantages:

- Has not been directly compared with mupirocin.
- Clinical effectiveness against methicillin-resistant isolates of Staphylococcus aureus has not been established.
- Indications are more limited (certain formulations of mupirocin are also indicated for the treatment of secondarily infected traumatic skin lesions, and for intranasal administration for the eradication of nasal colonization with methicillin-resistant S. aureus in adult patients and healthcare workers).
- Effectiveness and safety have been established in children as young as 9 months of age (compared with 2 months of age for mupirocin).

Most important risks/adverse events:

Unlikely to occur.

Most common adverse events:

Adults – application site irritation (2%), headache (2%); pediatric patients – application site pruritus (2%), pruritus (2%), diarrhea (2%), nasopharyngitis (2%).

Usual dosage:

A thin layer of ointment should be applied to the affected area twice a day for 5 days; the treated area may be covered with a sterile bandage or gauze dressing.

Product:

Ointment – 10 mg/gram (1%) in 5 gram, 10 gram, and 15 gram tubes.

Comments:

Retapamulin is the first of a new class of antibacterial agents designated as pleuromutilins. It is active against S. aureus and S. pyogenes, the bacteria that are most often responsible for causing impetigo, a highly contagious skin infection. Retapamulin inhibits bacterial protein synthesis through multiple mechanisms that differ from those of other antibacterial agents, including interacting at a site on the 50S subunit of the bacterial ribosome. Cross-resistance with other antibacterial agents has not been reported, but efficacy studies have not been done to determine its activity against strains of bacteria that are resistant to other antibacterial agents.

The effectiveness of retapamulin in the treatment of impetigo was demonstrated in a placebo-controlled study in which its clinical success rate was 86%. It has not been directly compared with mupirocin ointment. Although in vitro studies of retapamulin did not identify differences in susceptibility between methicillin-susceptible and methicillin-resistant isolates of S. aureus, the susceptibility did not correlate with clinical success rates in patients with methicillin-resistant S. aureus, and its indication for impetigo caused by S. aureus is limited to infection caused by methicillin-susceptible isolates.

Rilonacept (Arcalyst – Regeneron)
Agent for Cryopyrin-Associated Periodic Syndromes
2008

New Drug Comparison Rating = 5 (important advance)

Indication:

Administered subcutaneously for the treatment of Cryopyrin-Associated Periodic Syndromes (CAPS), including Familial Cold Autoinflammatory Syndrome (FCAS) and Muckle-Wells Syndrome (MWS) in adults and children 12 and older.

Comparable drugs:

None (Canakinumab [Ilaris] was subsequently marketed in 2009 for the treatment of CAPS).

Advantages:

• First drug to be demonstrated to be effective for the treatment of CAPS.

Disadvantages/Limitations:

• May interfere with the immune response and increase the risk of infections.

Most important risks/adverse events:

Increased risk of infection (treatment should not be initiated in patients who have an active or chronic infection; in patients being treated with rilonacept, therapy should be discontinued if a serious infection develops); concurrent use with a tumor necrosis factor (TNF) inhibitor (e.g., etanercept [Enbrel]) or the interleukin-1 (IL-1) blocker anakinra (Kineret) should be avoided because of the increased risk of infection; live vaccines should not be given to patients being treated with rilonacept, and patients should receive all recommended vaccinations before being treated with the drug.

Most common adverse events:

Injection-site reactions (48%), upper respiratory tract infections (26%), elevated blood lipid concentrations.

Usual dosage:

Administered subcutaneously into the left and right sides of the abdomen and the left and right thighs; in adult patients (18 years and above), treatment should be initiated with a loading dose of 320 mg delivered as two 2-mL injections of 160 mg each given on the same day at two different sites; treatment should be continued at weekly intervals at a dosage of 160 mg once a week as a single injection; in patients aged 12 to 17 years, the initial loading dose is 4.4 mg/kg, up to a maximum of 320 mg, delivered as one or

173

two injections with a maximum single-injection volume of 2 mL; treatment should be continued at weekly intervals at a dosage of 2.2 mg/kg, up to a maximum of 160 mg, once a week as a single injection.

Product:

Vials – 220 mg (should be stored in a refrigerator inside the original carton); contents of a vial should be reconstituted with 2.3 mL of preservative-free Sterile Water for Injection; vial should be shaken for one minute and then allowed to sit for one minute; resulting solution is viscous and contains the drug in a concentration of 80 mg/mL.

Comments:

CAPS are a group of rare, inherited chronic inflammatory diseases that are characterized, in part, by symptoms such as recurrent rash, fever/chills, joint pain, fatigue, and eye pain/redness. CAPS include three related disorders, FCAS, MWS, and neonatal-onset multisystem inflammatory disease (NOMID). The symptoms of FCAS are triggered by exposure to cooling temperatures, and MWS symptoms are triggered by random, unknown factors and possibly exercise, stress, and cold. It is often associated with hearing loss and/or amyloidosis. CAPS are generally caused by mutations in the NLRP-3 (nucleotide-binding domain, leucine-rich family [NLR], pyrin domain containing 3) gene, which encodes cryopyrin, a protein that regulates inflammation in the body. The mutation in the NLRP-3 gene causes increased activity of cryopyrin, which causes an overproduction of interleukin (IL)-1 beta, resulting in an inflammatory response and the symptoms of CAPS.

Rilonacept is a dimeric fusion protein consisting of the ligand-binding domains of the extracellular portions of the human IL-1 receptor component and IL-1 receptor accessory protein linked in-line to the Fc portion of human immunoglobulin G1. It acts as an IL-1 blocker. Rilonacept is the first drug to be approved for the treatment of CAPS and its effectiveness was demonstrated in a placebo-controlled study. Patients treated with the new drug experienced improvement of symptoms within several days following initiation of therapy. In 2009, canakinumab was marketed as the second drug to be approved for the treatment of CAPS.

Romiplostim (Nplate – Amgen)
Agent for Immune Thrombocytopenic Purpura
2008

New Drug Comparison Rating (NDCR) = 5 (important advance)

Indication:

Administered subcutaneously for the treatment of thrombocytopenia in patients with chronic immune (idiopathic) thrombocytopenic purpura (ITP) who have had an insufficient response to corticosteroids, immunoglobulins, or splenectomy; should be used only in patients with ITP whose degree of thrombocytopenia and clinical condition increase the risk of bleeding.

Comparable drugs:

None (subsequent to the marketing of romiplostim, eltrombopag [Promacta] was approved in late 2008 for the same indication).

Advantages:

- First drug to be demonstrated to be effective for the treatment of thrombocytopenia in patients with chronic ITP.
- Unique mechanism of action (a thrombopoietin receptor agonist).

Disadvantages/Limitations

- Increases the risk for reticulin deposition within the bone marrow.
- May increase the risk for hematological malignancies.
- Available only through a restricted distribution program.

Most important risks/adverse events:

Increases the risk of reticulin deposition in the bone marrow (that may increase the risk of bone marrow fibrosis); excessive doses may increase platelet count to a level that produces thrombotic/thromboembolic complications; may increase the risk for hematological malignancies; formation of neutralizing antibodies should be evaluated if platelet counts significantly decrease following an initial response to treatment; discontinuation of treatment may result in thrombocytopenia that is worse than that which was present prior to treatment; may cause fetal harm – Pregnancy Category C (women who are pregnant should be enrolled in a Pregnancy Registry).

Most common adverse events:

Headache (35%; placebo – 32%), arthralgia (26%; placebo – 20%), dizziness (17%), insomnia (16%), myalgia (14%), pain in extremity (13%), abdominal pain (11%).

Usual dosage:

Administered subcutaneously; initial dosage – 1 mcg/kg once a week; weekly dosage is adjusted by increments of 1 mcg/kg to achieve and maintain a platelet count of 50×10^9/liter or higher as necessary to reduce the risk for bleeding; maximum weekly dosage should not exceed 10 mcg/kg; should not be administered if platelet count is higher than 400×10^9/liter; treatment should be discontinued if the platelet count does not increase after 4 weeks at the maximum dosage.

Products:

Vials – 250 mcg, 500 mcg (should be stored in their carton in a refrigerator); should be reconstituted with preservative-free Sterile Water for Injection; vial should be gently swirled, but should not be shaken or vigorously agitated; reconstituted product should be protected from light; injection volume may be very small and a syringe with graduations to 0.01 mL should be used; available only through the restricted distribution program Nplate NEXUS in which physicians and patients must register.

Comments:

Chronic ITP is an autoimmune disorder characterized by low platelet counts, which may result in serious bleeding events. Romiplostim is an Fc-peptide fusion protein (peptibody; i.e., having characteristics of both peptides and antibodies) that is produced by recombinant DNA technology. It acts similarly to the naturally occurring protein thrombopoietin (TPO) and increases platelet production through binding and activation of TPO receptors. It is the first drug to be demonstrated to be effective for the treatment of thrombocytopenia in patients with chronic ITP. It was evaluated in two studies and the overall response rate with romiplostim was 83%, compared with 7% with placebo. Bleeding events were reduced by one-half in patients treated with romiplostim, and patients were often able to reduce or discontinue their concomitant ITP medications. In late 2008, eltrombopag was approved for the same indication (chronic ITP) as romiplostim. It also activates TPO receptors and is effective following oral administration.

Rotigotine (Neupro — Schwarz Pharma; UCB)

(Withdrawn from the market in April, 2008 because of the formation of rotigotine crystals in the patches)
Antiparkinson Agent
2007

New Drug Comparison Rating (NDCR) = 4 (significant advantages)

Indication:

For transdermal use for the treatment of the signs and symptoms of early-stage idiopathic Parkinson's disease.

Comparable drugs:

Pramipexole (Mirapex), ropinirole (Requip).

Advantages:

- Less frequent administration (once a day compared with three times a day for treating Parkinson's disease).
- Gradual release from transdermal formulation may result in less variation in concentration and clinical benefit.
- Gradual release from transdermal formulation may reduce the occurrence of adverse events that may be associated with peak concentrations multiple times a day with other agents.

Disadvantages:

- Has not been directly compared with pramipexole and ropinirole.
- Indications are more limited (pramipexole and ropinirole are also indicated for the treatment of advanced Parkinson's disease in conjunction with levodopa, as well as in the treatment of restless legs syndrome).
- Often causes application site reactions.
- Should not be used by patients with a history of hypersensitivity to sulfites.

Most important risks/adverse events:

Formulation contains sodium metabisulfite and should not be used in patients with a history of hypersensitivity to sulfites; falling asleep suddenly (sleep attacks) without warning and while engaged in normal activities; hallucinations; symptomatic hypotension and syncope; elevation of blood pressure and heart rate; weight gain and fluid retention; compulsive behaviors (e.g., urge to gamble); should not be applied to the same application site more often than once every 14 days; heat may increase the absorption of the drug and transdermal system should not be exposed to external sources of direct heat; backing layer contains aluminum and transdermal system should be removed prior to magnetic resonance imaging or cardioversion to avoid skin burns; action may be reduced by the concurrent use of a dopamine antagonist (e.g., antipsychotic agents).

Most common adverse events:

Application site reactions (37%), nausea (38%), somnolence (25%), dizziness (18%), headache (14%), vomiting (13%), insomnia (10%).

Usual dosage:

2 mg once a day (per 24 hours) initially and, based on clinical response and tolerability, the dosage may be increased weekly by 2 mg/24 hours to the maximum recommended dosage of 6 mg/24 hours; if it is necessary to discontinue treatment, the daily dosage should be reduced by 2 mg/24 hours every other day until the drug is completely withdrawn.

Products:

Transdermal systems (patches) – 2 mg/24 hours, 4 mg/24 hours, 6 mg/24 hours.

Comments:

Rotigotine appears to act primarily to stimulate dopamine D2 receptors in the brain, and its properties are most similar to those of pramipexole and ropinirole. These three agents are designated as non-ergoline dopamine agonists, whereas agents like bromocriptine (e.g., Parlodel) are ergot derivatives that may be associated with additional serious adverse events. Rotigotine is unique among the antiparkinson agents as it is the first to be supplied in a transdermal (patch) formulation for topical application. The gradual release of the medication from the transdermal formulation may provide more sustained clinical benefit and avoidance/reduction of some of the adverse events that may result from the peak concentrations that occur three times a day with the use of pramipexole and ropinirole. However, rotigotine has not been directly compared with these two agents in clinical studies; its effectiveness was demonstrated in placebo-controlled studies.

Rufinamide (Banzel – Eisai)
Antiepileptic Drug
2009

New Drug Comparison Rating (NDCR) = 4 (significant advantages)

Indication:

Adjunctive treatment of seizures associated with Lennox-Gastaut syndrome in children 4 years and older and adults.

Comparable drugs:

Lamotrigine (e.g., Lamictal), topiramate (e.g., Topamax), valproate (e.g., Depakote).

Advantages:

- Has reduced seizure frequency and seizure severity in some patients in whom previous treatment did not provide adequate seizure control.
- Has a labeled indication for Lennox-Gastaut syndrome (compared with valproate that, notwithstanding its common use in the treatment of this condition, does not have a labeled indication for this syndrome).
- Less likely to cause serious adverse events (lamotrigine has a boxed warning regarding serious rashes, valproate has a boxed warning regarding hepatotoxicity, pancreatitis, and teratogenicity, and topiramate may cause metabolic acidosis).
- Less risk if used during pregnancy (is in Pregnancy Category C compared with valproate that is in Category D).
- Less likely to interact with other drugs (compared with lamotrigine and valproate).

Disadvantages:

- Labeled indications are more limited (lamotrigine is also indicated for tonic-clonic seizures, partial seizures, and bipolar disorder, topiramate is also indicated for tonic-clonic seizures, partial seizures, and migraine prophylaxis, and valproate is indicated for partial seizures, absence seizures, acute manic or mixed episodes associated with bipolar disorder, and migraine prophylaxis).
- Use has not been evaluated in children less than 4 years of age (compared with lamotrigine and topiramate that are indicated for use in children as young as 2 years of age).
- May cause shortening of the QT interval of the electrocardiogram and is contraindicated in patients with Familial Short QT syndrome.
- Is administered twice a day (compared with certain formulations of valproate that may be administered once a day).
- Is not available in a formulation (e.g., liquid, chewable tablet) to facilitate administration in children.

Most important risks/adverse events:

Suicidal ideation and behavior (patients should be monitored for the emergence or worsening of depression, suicidal thoughts, and/or unusual changes in mood or behavior); central nervous system (CNS) effects (e.g., somnolence, fatigue, dizziness, coordination abnormalities, ataxia; patients should be advised not to engage in potentially hazardous activities until they have assessed whether the drug adversely affects their mental and/or motor performance, and

179

cautioned about the added risk if other CNS depressants, including alcoholic beverages, are used concurrently); shortening of the QT interval (contraindicated in patients with Familial Short QT syndrome); multiorgan hypersensitivity reactions (e.g., urticaria, hepatitis).

Most common adverse events:

In children, somnolence (17%), vomiting (17%), headache (16%), fatigue (9%), dizziness (8%), nausea (7%).

Usual dosage:

Should be administered with food; children 4 years and older – initial dosage of approximately 10 mg/kg/day in two equally divided doses; may be increased by approximately 10 mg/kg/day increments every other day to a target dosage of 45 mg/kg/day or 3200 mg/day, whichever is less, administered in two equally divided doses; adults – initial dosage of 400 – 800 mg/day in two equally divided doses; may be increased by 400 – 800 mg/day every 2 days until a maximum daily dosage of 3200 mg/day, in two equally divided doses, is reached; if treatment is to be discontinued, should be done gradually by reducing the dose by approximately 25% every 2 days.

Products:

Tablets – 200 mg, 400 mg; tablets are scored on both sides and may be cut in half for dosing flexibility; however, tablets do not readily provide the exact mg/kg dosage that has been calculated for use in children, and these dosages have been designated as "approximate".

Comments:

Lennox-Gastaut syndrome is a severe form of childhood epilepsy that is characterized by frequent episodes of multiple types of seizures such as atypical absence seizures, tonic seizures, and atonic seizures in which the patient has a loss of muscle tone and falls suddenly (a "drop attack"). Valproate is often considered the drug of first-choice although Lennox-Gastaut syndrome is not a labeled indication for its use. Treatment usually requires a multiple-antiepileptic drug (AED) regimen and the AEDs with labeled indications for this syndrome include lamotrigine, topiramate, and felbamate (Felbatol), with the latter agent being withheld for use for patients who do not adequately respond to other therapies because of the risks of aplastic anemia and liver failure.

Rufinamide is structurally unrelated to other AEDs and is thought to act by prolonging the inactive state of sodium channels. Its effectiveness was demonstrated in a placebo-controlled study in patients who were already taking one to three AEDs that were providing inadequate seizure control. In the patients in whom the new drug was added to their AED regimen there was a 33% decrease in total seizure frequency per 28 days and a 43% decrease in tonic-clonic seizure frequency per 28 days, compared with a 12% decrease and 1% decrease, respectively, in the patients in whom placebo was added to their AED regimen. In addition, there was improvement in the seizure severity rating in 53% of the patients receiving rufinamide, compared with 31% of those receiving placebo.

Like other AEDs, rufinamide may increase the risk of suicidal thoughts or behavior, and patients should be closely monitored. CNS effects (e.g., somnolence, fatigue) are common and patients should be cautioned about the pertinent risks. The concentration of rufinamide is decreased by the concurrent use of carbamazepine (e.g., Tegretol), phenobarbital, phenytoin (e.g., Dilantin), and primidone (e.g., Mysoline). Conversely, its concentration is increased by up to 70% when valproate is used concurrently. When treatment with either one of these agents is to be started in a patient who is already stabilized on the other agent, a lower dosage of the drug should be used when initiating treatment. Rufinamide may reduce the effectiveness of hormonal contraceptives and women using these products should be advised to use additional non-hormonal forms of contraception.

Sapropterin dihydrochloride (Kuvan – BioMarin)
Agent for Phenylketonuria
2007

New Drug Comparison Rating (NDCR) = 5 (important advance)

Indication:

To reduce blood phenylalanine concentrations in patients with hyperphenylalaninemia due to tetrahydrobiopterin- (BH4-) responsive phenylketonuria; used in conjunction with a phenylalanine-restricted diet.

Comparable drugs:

None.

Advantages:

• First drug to be approved for the reduction of phenylalanine concentrations for patients with phenylketonuria.

Disadvantages:

• Only available through a restricted distribution program.

Most important risks/adverse events:

Blood phenylalanine concentrations should be monitored during treatment; women who are treated with the drug during pregnancy are encouraged to enroll in a patient registry; should be used with caution in patients who are also being treated with drugs that inhibit folate metabolism (e.g., methotrexate), drugs that affect nitric oxide-mediated vasorelaxation (e.g., PDE-5 inhibitors [sildenafil (Viagra), tadalafil (Cialis), vardenafil (Levitra)]), and levodopa.

Most common adverse events:

Headache (15%), upper respiratory tract infection (12%), rhinorrhea (11%), pharyngolaryngeal pain (10%), diarrhea (8%), vomiting (8%), cough (7%).

Usual dosage:

10 mg/kg /day administered once a day; should be administered with food to increase absorption; dosage may be adjusted within the range of 5 to 20 mg/kg/day based on the response to therapy (i.e., blood phenylalanine concentrations).

Product:

Tablets – 100 mg; tablets should be dissolved in 120-240 mL of water or apple juice and administered within 15 minutes.

Comments:

Phenylketonuria (PKU) is an inherited disorder in which the activity of the enzyme phenylalanine hydroxylase (PAH) is deficient. PAH helps break down phenylalanine in the body and, when there is a deficiency of this enzyme, the increase in blood concentrations of phenylalanine results in an increased risk of neurologic and other problems. Tetrahydrobiopterin (BH4) is a cofactor for PAH, without which PAH does not function properly. Sapropterin is a synthetic form of BH4 that can activate residual PAH and decrease phenylalanine concentrations in some patients. Not all patients with PKU will respond to sapropterin and, in clinical trials, 20% to 56% of patients responded to treatment (BH4-responsive PKU). It is not possible to predict which patients will respond to sapropterin and the only way to know if a patient will respond is to initiate treatment with the medication and monitor blood phenylalanine concentrations. Patients who are treated with sapropterin must still be managed with a low-phenylalanine diet, and should have regular monitoring of blood phenylalanine concentrations.

Saxagliptin hydrochloride (Onglyza – Bristol-Myers Squibb; AstraZeneca)
Antidiabetic Agent
2009

New Drug Comparison Rating (NDCR) = 3 (no or minor advantages/disadvantages)

Indication:
As monotherapy or in combination regimens as an adjunct to diet and exercise to improve glycemic control in adults with type 2 diabetes mellitus.

Comparable drug:
Sitagliptin (Januvia).

Advantages:
- May be less likely to cause hypersensitivity reactions.

Disadvantages:
- Has not been directly compared with sitagliptin in clinical studies.
- Is more likely to interact with CYP3A4/5 inhibitors.
- May be more likely to decrease absolute lymphocyte counts (clinical significance has not been determined).
- Not available in combination formulations with metformin.

Most important risks/adverse events:
Risk of hypoglycemia when used in combination with a sulfonylurea or other insulin secretagogues (a lower dosage of the sulfonylurea may be required); action may be increased by the concurrent use of a strong CYP3A4/5 inhibitor (e.g., clarithromycin [e.g., Biaxin]); is primarily eliminated in the urine and the dosage should be reduced in patients with moderate or severe renal impairment.

Most common adverse events:
Upper respiratory tract infection (8%), urinary tract infection (7%), headache (7%).

Usual dosage:
5 mg once a day; a dosage of 2.5 mg once a day is recommended in patients also being treated with a strong CYP3A4/5 inhibitor, and in patients with moderate or severe renal impairment or end-stage renal disease requiring hemodialysis; is removed by hemodialysis and should be administered following hemodialysis.

Products:
Tablets – 2.5 mg, 5 mg.

Comments:

Incretins are naturally occurring hormones that increase insulin secretion in the presence of elevated glucose concentrations (e.g., following meals). They are rapidly inactivated by the enzyme dipeptidyl peptidase-4 (DPP-4). Sitagliptin and saxagliptin are DPP-4 inhibitors that slow the inactivation of incretins, thereby increasing and prolonging their action. Saxagliptin is primarily metabolized via the CYP3A4/5 pathways to an active metabolite, 5-hydroxy saxagliptin, that is also a DPP-4 inhibitor with approximately one-half the potency of the parent compound.

When used as monotherapy, saxagliptin reduced glycosylated hemoglobin (A1C) by approximately 0.6% compared with placebo and, when used with metformin, a thiazolidinedione (pioglitazone [Actos], rosiglitazone [Avandia]), or glyburide, reduced A1C by approximately this same percentage compared with placebo plus the other drug.

Saxagliptin is well tolerated and the incidence of adverse events reported in the clinical studies was generally similar to that with placebo. When used in combination with a thiazolidinedione, peripheral edema was experienced more frequently (8%) than in the patients receiving placebo instead of the new drug (4%). The DPP-4 inhibitors do not cause hypoglycemia; however, their concurrent use with an agent known to cause hypoglycemia (e.g., a sulfonylurea) should be closely monitored. There have been infrequent reposts of serious hypersensitivity reactions in the postmarketing experience with sitagliptin, and saxagliptin may be less likely to cause such events. Although weight gain is sometimes associated with certain antidiabetic agents, significant changes in weight have not been experienced with saxagliptin. The new drug is more likely than sitagliptin to interact with strong CYP3A4/5 inhibitors.

Silodosin (Rapaflo – Watson)
Agent for Benign Prostatic Hyperplasia
2009

New Drug Comparison Rating (NDCR) = 3 (no or minor advantages/disadvantages)

Indication:

Treatment of the signs and symptoms of benign prostatic hyperplasia.

Comparable drugs:

Tamsulosin (Flomax), alfuzosin (Uroxatral), doxazosin (e.g., Cardura XL), terazosin (e.g., Hytrin).

Advantages:

- Convenient dosage regimen that does not require dosage titration (compared with tamsulosin, doxazosin, and terazosin).
- Less likely to cause a reduction in blood pressure (compared with doxazosin and terazosin).
- Has not been associated with prolongation of the QT interval of the electrocardiogram (compared with alfuzosin).
- May be used in patients with moderate hepatic impairment (compared with alfuzosin that is contraindicated in patients with moderate or severe hepatic impairment).
- Has not been associated with reactions in patients who are allergic to sulfonamides (compared with tamsulosin with which there have been rare reports of such reactions).
- Has not been associated with interactions with cimetidine (compared with tamsulosin).

Disadvantages:

- Studies that directly compare silodosin with similar agents are limited.
- Labeled indication is more limited (compared with tamsulosin that has also been approved for concurrent use with dutasteride [Avodart]).
- Is contraindicated in patients with severe renal impairment.
- Is contraindicated in patients who are also being treated with a strong CYP3A4 inhibitor (compared with tamsulosin, doxazosin, and terazosin).
- Concurrent use with strong P-glycoprotein inhibitors (e.g., cyclosporine [e.g., Neoral]) is not recommended.
- More likely to cause retrograde/abnormal ejaculation (compared with alfuzosin, doxazosin, and terazosin).

Most important risks/adverse events:

Contraindicated in patients with severe renal impairment, severe hepatic impairment, and in patients being treated with a strong CYP3A4 inhibitor (e.g., clarithromycin [e.g., Biaxin]); postural hypotension; intraoperative floppy iris syndrome (caution must be observed during cataract surgery); should not be used concurrently with other alpha-adrenergic blocking agents.

185

Most common adverse events:

Retrograde/abnormal ejaculation (28%); orthostatic hypotension (3%), dizziness (3%), diarrhea (3%).

Usual dosage:

8 mg once a day with a meal; in patients with moderate renal impairment, 4 mg once a day with a meal.

Products:

Capsules – 4 mg, 8 mg.

Comments:

Silodosin is the fifth alpha-1-adrenergic receptor antagonist (alpha-blockers) to be approved for the treatment of the signs and symptoms of benign prostatic hyperplasia (BPH). Its properties and actions are most similar to those of tamsulosin.. The effectiveness of silodosin was demonstrated in two placebo-controlled studies which evaluated irritative (e.g., frequency, urgency) and obstructive (e.g., hesitancy) symptoms. The results of one study in Japan reported that silodosin was more effective than placebo and not inferior to tamsulosin, although the latter agent was used in a lower dosage (0.2 mg once a day) than is generally used in the United States (0.4 mg once a day). The alpha-blockers often are used concurrently with finasteride (Proscar) or dutasteride (Avodart) to reduce the symptoms of BPH via two mechanisms of action. In 2008, the FDA approved the use of tamsulosin and dutasteride in combination; however, studies of the use of silodosin with finasteride or dutasteride have not been conducted.

Sinecatechins (Veregen – PharmaDerm)
Agent for Genital Warts
2008

New Drug Comparison Rating (NDCR) = 2 (significant disadvantages)

Indication:

Topical treatment of external genital and perianal warts in immunocompetent patients 18 years and older.

Comparable drugs:

Self-applied medications for genital warts: imiquimod (Aldara), podofilox (Condylox).

Advantages:

- Different mechanism of action.
- May be less likely to cause systemic adverse events (compared with imiquimod).
- Does not have a limitation on the area of wart tissue to be treated or the amount of formulation used (compared with podofilox).

Disadvantages:

- Has not been directly compared with other agents in clinical studies.
- Labeled indications are more limited (compared with imiquimod that also has labeled indications for actinic keratosis and superficial basal cell carcinoma).
- Must be applied more frequently (three times a day compared with three times a week with imiquimod and twice a day for three consecutive days in each weekly cycle with podofilox).
- May weaken condoms and vaginal diaphragms.
- May stain clothing and bedding.

Most important risks/adverse events:

Use on open wounds should be avoided.

Most common adverse events:

Erythema (70%), pruritus (69%), burning (67%), pain/discomfort (56%), erosion/ulceration (49%), edema (45%), induration (35%), vesicular rash (20%).

Usual dosage:

A strand of ointment (approximately 0.5 cm) is applied three times a day to all external genital and perianal warts, leaving a thin layer of the ointment on the warts; treatment should be continued until the warts have completely cleared, but not for a period longer than 16 weeks; treated areas should not be covered or wrapped as to be occlusive.

187

Product:

Ointment – 15%; should be stored in a refrigerator prior to dispensing.

Comments:

Genital warts (condyloma acuminata) are caused by the human papillomavirus (HPV). HPV infection is highly contagious and is one of the most common sexually-transmitted diseases. Epidemiologic data also identify an increased incidence of cervical cancer associated with the virus. Sinecatechins is a botanical product that is a partially purified fraction of an extract of green tea leaves that contains a mixture of catechins and other green tea components. Catechins constitute 85 to 95% of the total drug substance which includes more than 55% of epigallocatechin gallate. The product has been approved for the topical treatment of external genital and perianal warts; its mechanism of action has not been specifically identified although it has demonstrated antioxidant activity in vitro.

The effectiveness of sinecatechins ointment has been demonstrated in two studies in which it was compared with the ointment vehicle. Complete clearance of warts was experienced by 54% of patients, compared with 35% of those who received the vehicle. The median time to complete clearance of the warts was 16 weeks and 10 weeks in the two studies. The rate of recurrence of warts 12 weeks following completion of treatment in patients with complete clearance was 7% for those treated with sinecatechins and 6% for those treated with the vehicle. The product has not been evaluated for the treatment of urethral, intra-vaginal, cervical, rectal, or intra-anal HPV disease, or in immunosuppressed patients.

Approximately two-thirds of the patients treated with sinecatechins experienced either a moderate or severe adverse reaction that resulted in discontinuation or interruption of treatment in 5% of patients. The ointment may weaken condoms and vaginal diaphragms, and concurrent use, as well as sexual contact while the ointment is on the skin, is not recommended. The ointment may stain clothing and bedding.

Sitagliptin phosphate (Januvia – Merck)
Antidiabetic Agent
2006

New Drug Comparison Rating (NDCR) = 4 (significant advantages)

Indications:

As an adjunct to diet and exercise to improve glycemic control in patients with type 2 diabetes mellitus; used as monotherapy or in combination with metformin or a thiazolidinedione when the single agent alone, with diet and exercise, does not provide adequate glycemic control; (additional experience in combination with other antidiabetic agents [e.g., sulfonylureas] has resulted in revision of indication to delete mention of specific other agents with which it is used in combination).

Comparable drugs:

Exenatide (Byetta), metformin (e.g., Glucophage), pioglitazone (Actos), rosiglitazone (Avandia); (another comparable drug, saxagliptin [Onglyza] has been subsequently marketed).

Advantages:

- Has a unique mechanism of action (inhibition of dipeptidyl peptidase-4).
- Less likely to cause adverse events (e.g., less likely than exenatide and metformin to cause gastrointestinal effects; less likely than pioglitazone and rosiglitazone to cause edema and weight gain).
- Less likely to interact with other drugs.
- May be used in patients with renal impairment (with adjustment of dosage; compared with metformin that is contraindicated).
- May be used in patients with congestive heart failure (compared with metformin that is contraindicated in patients requiring treatment for congestive heart failure).
- Is administered orally (compared with exenatide that is administered subcutaneously).
- Is in Pregnancy Category B (compared with exenatide, pioglitazone, and rosiglitazone that are in Category C).

Disadvantages:

- May reduce hemoglobin A1C to a lesser extent than the other agents.
- Indications are more limited (e.g., compared with metformin, pioglitazone, and rosiglitazone that are also indicated for use in combination with sulfonylureas and insulin); (indications have subsequently expanded).
- Not available in combination formulations with other antidiabetic agents (compared with metformin, pioglitazone, and rosiglitazone); (subsequently marketed in a combination with metformin [Janumet]).

Most important risks/adverse events:

Risk of hypoglycemia when used in combination with a sulfonylurea and a lower dosage of the sulfonylurea may be required; is primarily excreted in the urine in unchanged form and dosage should be reduced in patients with renal impairment; hypersensitivity reactions. A warning about a risk of pancreatitis has been subsequently added to the labeling.

Most common adverse events:

Upper respiratory tract infection (6%), nasopharyngitis (5%), headache (5%); (hepatic enzyme elevations have been reported in the postmarketing experience).

Usual dosage:

100 mg once a day; dosage should be reduced in patients with renal impairment.

Products:

Tablets – 25 mg, 50 mg, 100 mg; (subsequently marketed in a combination formulation with metformin [Janumet]. 50 mg/500 mg, 50 mg/1000 mg).

Comments:

In 2005, exenatide was marketed as the first agent for the treatment of diabetes that acts by increasing the action of incretins. The incretins are rapidly inactivated by the enzyme dipeptidyl peptidase-4 (DPP-4). Sitagliptin is a DPP-4 inhibitor that is administered orally and slows the inactivation of incretins, thereby increasing and prolonging their action. When used as monotherapy, sitagliptin reduced hemoglobin A1C by 0.6% to 0.8% compared with placebo and, when used with metformin or pioglitazone, reduced A1C by approximately this same percentage compared to the placebo plus metformin or pioglitazone regimens.

The use of some antidiabetic agents (e.g., sulfonylureas, thiazolidinediones) has been associated with weight gain, whereas the use of exenatide has been associated with weight loss. In the studies of sitagliptin, there was no or little change in body weight compared with baseline.

A second DPP-4 inhibitor, saxagliptin (Onglyza) was marketed in 2009.

Solifenacin succinate (Vesicare – Astellas; GlaxoSmithKline)
Agent for Overactive Bladder
2005

New Drug Comparison Rating (NDCR) = 3 (no or minor advantages/disadvantages)

Indication:
Treatment of overactive bladder with symptoms of urge urinary incontinence, urgency, and urinary frequency.

Comparable drugs:
Darifenacin (Enablex), oxybutynin (e.g., Ditropan XL), tolterodine (Detrol LA), trospium (Sanctura).

Advantages:
• Administered once a day (compared with trospium that is administered twice a day).

Disadvantages:
• May cause QT interval prolongation.

Most important risks/adverse events:
Contraindicated in patients with urinary retention, gastric retention, or uncontrolled narrow-angle glaucoma, and in patients who are at risk of these conditions; QT interval prolongation; is extensively metabolized (primarily via the CYP3A4 pathway) and its action may be significantly increased by the concurrent use of a potent CYP3A4 inhibitor (e.g., clarithromycin [e.g., Biaxin]); not recommended for use in patients with severe hepatic impairment.

Most common adverse events:
Dry mouth (11%), constipation (5%), blurred vision (4%)—incidences reported are with a dosage of 5 mg once a day and are higher with a dosage of 10 mg once a day.

Usual dosage:
5 mg once a day, initially; if satisfactorily tolerated, may be increased to 10 mg once a day; dosage should not exceed 5 mg once a day in patients with moderate hepatic impairment or severe renal impairment, or in patients also being treated with a potent CYP3A4 inhibitor.

Products:
Tablets – 5 mg, 10 mg.

Comments:

Solifenacin has been suggested to have a selective action on the muscarinic receptors involved in bladder contraction. However, its efficacy and incidence of anticholinergic adverse events do not distinguish it from the other agents used in the treatment of overactive bladder. Most of the adverse events and precautions associated with its use are related to its anticholinergic activity. Concurrent use with another agent having anticholinergic activity (e.g., diphenhydramine [e.g., Benadryl]) may increase the severity of anticholinergic adverse events.

Unlike the other agents used in the treatment of overactive bladder, the labeling for solifenacin includes a precaution regarding use in patients with congenital or acquired QT prolongation. Prolongation of the QT interval appears unlikely even with the use of the maximum recommended dosage of solifenacin (10 mg once a day), but this possibility should be considered in patients who are at risk (e.g., those taking an antiarrhythmic agent).

Sorafenib tosylate (Nexavar – Bayer; Onyx)
Antineoplastic Agent
2006

New Drug Comparison Rating (NDCR) = 4 (significant advantages)

Indication:
Treatment of patients with advanced renal cell carcinoma; (subsequently approved for the treatment of unresectable hepatocellular carcinoma).

Comparable drug (that is indicated for renal cell carcinoma):
Aldesleukin (Proleukin); (four other comparable drugs, sunitinib [Sutent], pazopanib [Votrient], temsirolimus [Torisel], and everolimus [Afinitor], have been subsequently marketed for the treatment of renal cell carcinoma).

Advantages:
- May be effective in some patients who do not respond to or cannot tolerate aldesleukin.
- Is less likely to cause serious adverse events.
- Is administered orally (aldesleukin is administered intravenously).

Disadvantages:
- May interact with more medications.
- Available only through a restricted distribution program.

Most important risks/adverse events:
Cardiac ischemia and/or infarction; hypertension; hemorrhage (concurrent use with warfarin must be closely monitored); wound healing complications (treatment should be interrupted in patients undergoing major surgical procedures); dermatologic toxicity (e.g., hand-foot skin reaction, rash); may cause harm to a fetus and should not be used during pregnancy; action may be reduced by the concurrent use of a CYP3A4 inducer (e.g., rifampin [e.g., Rifadin]); inhibits glucuronidation via the UGT1A1 and UGT1A9 pathways and may increase the action of irinotecan (Camptosar) and doxorubicin (e.g., Adriamycin) that are substrates for these metabolic pathways;.

Most common adverse events:
Diarrhea (43%), rash (40%), fatigue (37%), hand-foot skin reactions (30%), alopecia (27%), nausea (23%), pruritus (19%), hypertension (17%), hemorrhage (15%), neuropathy-sensory effects (13%), hypophosphatemia (45%), elevated lipases (41%), lymphopenia (23%).

Usual dosage:

400 mg twice a day at least 1 hour before or 2 hours after eating.

Product:

Tablets – 200 mg.

Comments:

Sorafenib is a multikinase inhibitor that interacts with multiple intracellular and cell surface kinases and specifically targets several serine/threonine and receptor tyrosine kinases. The properties of sorafenib are most similar to those of erlotinib (Tarceva). Both drugs decrease tumor cell proliferation, but sorafenib appears to also inhibit angiogenesis.

Sorafenib is only the second drug to be approved for the treatment of advanced renal cell carcinoma, joining aldesleukin that was first marketed in 1992. It may be used as a first-line treatment or in patients who have not responded adequately to or have not tolerated other therapies. In the largest study, the median progression-free survival was 167 days in the patients receiving sorafenib, compared with 84 days in the patients randomized to placebo. In an interim survival analysis, overall survival was longer for sorafenib than placebo, but the results did not meet the prespecified criteria for statistical significance.

Since the time sorafenib was marketed in early 2006, four other drugs have been marketed for the treatment of renal cell carcinoma. Sunitinib (Sutent) was marketed later in 2006, temsirolimus (Torisel) in 2007, and everolimus [Afinitor] and pazopanib [Votrient] in 2009.

Sunitinib malate (Sutent –Pfizer)
Antineoplastic Agent
2006

New Drug Comparison Rating (NDCR) = 4 (significant advantages)

Indications:

Treatment of gastrointestinal stromal tumor (GIST) after disease progression on or intolerance to imatinib; treatment of advanced renal cell carcinoma.

Comparable drugs:

Sorafenib (Nexavar – with respect to use for advanced renal cell carcinoma), imatinib (Gleevec – with respect to use for GIST); (other comparable drugs [with respect to use in patients with renal cell carcinoma], temsirolimus [Torisel], everolimus [Afinitor], and pazopanib [Votrient] have subsequently been marketed).

Advantages:

- May be effective in some patients with renal cell carcinoma who do not respond to or tolerate other therapies.
- May be effective in some patients with GIST who do not respond to or tolerate imatinib.

Disadvantages:

- Is not indicated for first-line treatment of GIST.
- May cause discoloration of skin.

Most important risks/adverse events:

Decreased left ventricular ejection fraction (use in patients with cardiac risk factors should be carefully evaluated); hemorrhage; hypertension; neutropenia/anemia/thrombocytopenia (complete blood counts and platelet counts should be performed at the beginning of each treatment cycle); thyroid dysfunction; QT interval prolongation and torsades de pointes (warning added to labeling subsequent to initial marketing); may cause harm to a fetus and should not be used during pregnancy; is extensively metabolized, primarily via the CYP3A4 pathway, and action may be increased by the concurrent use of CYP3A4 inhibitors (e.g., clarithromycin [e.g., Biaxin]), and decreased by the concurrent use of CYP3A4 inducers (e.g., rifampin [e.g., Rifadin]); the CYP3A4 inducer St. John's wort should not be used concurrently.

Most common adverse events (incidence in patients with renal cell carcinoma):

Fatigue (74%), diarrhea (55%), nausea (54%), mucositis/stomatitis (53%), dyspepsia (46%), altered taste (43%), rash (38%), vomiting (37%), skin discoloration (33% - possibly attributed to the yellow color of the drug), anorexia (31%), elevations in liver enzymes.

Usual dosage:

50 mg once a day on a schedule of 4 weeks on treatment followed by 2 weeks off treatment; if it is not possible to avoid concurrent use of a strong CYP3A4 inhibitor, a dosage reduction to a minimum of 37.5 mg daily should be considered; a dosage increase to a maximum of 87.5 mg daily should be considered if a CYP3A4 inducer is to be used concurrently.

Products:

Tablets – 12.5 mg, 25 mg, 50 mg; (a capsule formulation in a 37.5 mg potency has been subsequently approved).

Comments:

Sunitinib is a multikinase inhibitor that primarily acts at receptor tyrosine kinases, some of which are implicated in tumor growth, pathologic angiogenesis, and metastatic progression of cancer. Its properties are most similar to those of sorafenib, another multikinase inhibitor that was marketed earlier in 2006 for the treatment of advanced renal cell carcinoma. It is also compared with imatinib with respect to their use in the treatment of gastrointestinal stromal tumor (GIST), a rare stomach cancer. Imatinib is the recommended treatment for GIST but the benefit from this treatment may be limited and/or of short duration, and some patients are not able to tolerate imatinib. In two studies in patients with GIST, the median time to tumor progression was 27 weeks in those receiving sunitinib compared with 6 weeks for the patients receiving placebo. Sunitinib has not been directly compared with imatinib in clinical studies.

Sunitinib is the third drug to be approved for the treatment of advanced renal cell carcinoma, joining aldesleukin (Proleukin) and sorafenib. Additional drugs including temsirolimus, everolimus, and pazopanib have been subsequently marketed, and bevacizumab (Avastin) has been approved for use in combination with interferon alfa.

Tapentadol hydrochloride (Nucynta – PriCara)
Analgesic
2009

New Drug Comparison Rating (NDCR) = 3 (no or minor advantages/disadvantages)

Indication:
For the relief of moderate to severe acute pain in patients 18 years of age and older.

Comparable drugs:
Oxycodone (e.g., OxyIR), tramadol (e.g., Ultram).

Advantages:
- Relieves pain by more than one mechanism of action (compared with oxycodone).
- Has a stronger analgesic action (compared with tramadol).
- Is less likely to cause gastrointestinal adverse events (compared with oxycodone).
- May be less likely to cause seizures and serotonin syndrome (compared with tramadol).
- Is less likely to interact with other medications (compared with tramadol).

Disadvantages:
- Labeled indication is limited to the relief of acute pain and is not indicated for use over extended periods (e.g., for chronic pain).
- Greater risk of dependence and abuse and is classified in Schedule II (compared with tramadol that is not a controlled substance).
- Is not available in a controlled-release formulation and must be administered more frequently than the controlled-release formulations of oxycodone and tramadol.

Most important risks/adverse events:
Contraindicated in patients with impaired pulmonary function or paralytic ileus, or concurrently with or within 14 days of a monoamine oxidase inhibitor; respiratory depression (risk is increased in elderly, debilitated patients); elevated intracranial pressure (e.g., increased risk in patients with head injuries); potential for dependence and abuse (classified in Schedule II); central nervous system depressant (CNS) effects (patients should be advised to exercise caution when engaged in potentially hazardous activities, and of the additive effects of other CNS depressants, including alcoholic beverages); seizures (must be used with caution in patients with a history of seizures); serotonin syndrome (in patients also being treated with serotonergic medications); must be used with caution in patients with biliary tract disease, including acute pancreatitis; should not be used during or immediately prior to labor and delivery; should not be used by a nursing mother.

Most common adverse events:

Nausea (30%), vomiting (18%), dizziness (24%), somnolence (15%).

Usual dosage:

Initiate treatment with a dosage of 50 mg, 75 mg, or 100 mg depending upon pain intensity; second dose may be administered as soon as one hour after the first dose if adequate pain relief is not attained with the first dose; subsequent doses are administered every 4 to 6 hours; daily doses greater than 700 mg on the first day of therapy and 600 mg on subsequent days have not been studied and are not recommended; in patients with moderate hepatic impairment, the recommended initial dosage is 50 mg with the interval between doses no less than 8 hours; in elderly patients, consideration should also be given to starting treatment with a dose of 50 mg.

Products:

Tablets – 50 mg, 75 mg, 100 mg.

Comments:

Tapentadol is a centrally-acting analgesic that, like the opioid analgesics (e.g., oxycodone), is a mu-opioid receptor agonist, but it also inhibits norepinephrine reuptake. Its pharmacological actions are most similar to those of tramadol that has an opioid agonist action and also inhibits norepinephrine and serotonin reuptake. However, the opioid agonist action of the new drug is stronger than that of tramadol, and the analgesic benefit of a dose of 100 mg of tapentadol is similar to that provided by a 15 mg dose of oxycodone. Tapentadol also has a greater potential for dependence and abuse than tramadol and is classified in Schedule II, whereas tramadol is not a controlled substance.

In contrast to tramadol, tapentadol is metabolized to only a limited extent via cytochrome P450 metabolic pathways and is not likely to interact with other medications via pharmacokinetic mechanisms.

Telavancin (Vibativ – Astellas)
Antibiotic
2009

New Drug Comparison Rating (NDCR) = 3 (no or minor advantages/disadvantages)

Indications:

Administered via intravenous infusion for the treatment of adult patients with complicated skin and skin structure infections (cSSSI) caused by susceptible isolates of the following Gram-positive bacteria: Staphylococcus aureus (including methicillin-susceptible and –resistant isolates), Streptococcus pyogenes, Streptococcus agalactiae, Streptococcus anginosus group (includes S. anginosus, S. intermedius, and S. constellatus), or Enterococcus faecalis (vancomycin-susceptible isolates only).

Comparable drug:

Vancomycin.

Advantages:

- May be effective in some Gram-positive infections that are resistant to other antibiotics.
- May have a lower risk of ototoxicity.
- Administered once a day (whereas vancomycin is often administered every 12 hours).
- Does not require monitoring of serum concentrations.

Disadvantages:

- Fewer labeled indications (vancomycin is also indicated for infections at other sites including endocarditis).
- Greater risk of fetal harm if used during pregnancy.
- Use has not been evaluated in pediatric patients.
- May cause QT interval prolongation.
- More likely to cause taste disturbance, nausea, and vomiting.
- Interferes with certain tests used to monitor coagulation (e.g., prothrombin time, international normalized ratio [INR]).

Most important risks/adverse events:

Risk of fetal harm (boxed warning; Pregnancy Category C; women of childbearing potential should have a serum pregnancy test performed prior to administration); nephrotoxicity (renal function [i.e., serum creatinine, creatinine clearance] should be monitored [at 48- to 72-hour intervals during treatment or more frequently if clinically indicated]; in patients with renal dysfunction, the solubilizer hydroxypropyl-beta-cyclodextrin may accumulate); infusion-related reactions (excessive rate of infusion may result in "red-man syndrome" [i.e., flushing of the upper body, urticaria, rash]); QT interval prolongation (caution must be exercised in patients with risk factors [e.g., also

199

taking other medications known to cause QT prolongation]); Clostridium difficile-associated diarrhea; coagulation test interference (e.g., prothrombin time, INR [blood samples should be collected as close as possible prior to the patient's next dose]).

Most common adverse events:

Taste disturbance (33%), nausea (27%), vomiting (14%), foamy urine (13%).

Usual dosage:

Administered via intravenous infusion over 60 minutes; 10 mg/kg once every 24 hours for 7 to 14 days; dosage should be reduced in patients with impaired renal function.

Products:

Single-use vials – 250 mg, 750 mg; should be stored in a refrigerator; should be reconstituted with 5% Dextrose Injection, Sterile Water for Injection, or 0.9% Sodium Chloride Injection.

Comments:

Telavancin is a lipoglycopeptide that is a synthetic derivative of vancomycin. Other antibiotics that are used in the treatment of serious/complicated infections caused by Gram-positive bacteria (e.g., staphylococci) include nafcillin, oxacillin, linezolid (Zyvox), daptomycin (Cubicin), tigecycline (Tygacil), and quinupristin/dalfopristin (Synercid). Telavancin was evaluated in studies in patients with cSSSI in which it was compared with vancomycin. The two antibiotics were generally similar in their effectiveness, although the clinical cure rates for telavancin were lower in patients 65 years of age and older (compared with those less than 65) and in patients with a creatinine clearance of 50 mL/minute or less. Reduced cure rates of the same magnitude were not observed in patients receiving vancomycin.

Telbivudine (Tyzeka – Idenix; Novartis)
Antiviral Agent
2006

New Drug Comparison Rating (NDCR) = 3 (no or minor advantages/disadvantages)

Indication:
Treatment of chronic hepatitis B virus (HBV) infection in adults with evidence of active viral replication and either evidence of persistent elevations in serum aminotransferases (ALT or AST) or histologically active disease.

Comparable drugs:
Adefovir dipivoxil (Hepsera), entecavir (Baraclude), lamivudine (Epivir-HBV); (indications for tenofovir [Viread] have subsequently been expanded to include chronic HBV infection).

Advantages:
- May be more effective in reducing viral load (compared with lamivudine and adefovir).
- Is not likely to reduce the effectiveness of antiviral agents used to treat HIV infection in patients who are co-infected with HBV and HIV (compared with lamivudine and adefovir).
- Is in Pregnancy Category B (other drugs are in Category C).

Disadvantages:
- May be more likely to cause musculoskeletal effects (e.g., myopathy).
- Not indicated in patients less than 16 years of age (compared with lamivudine that is indicated for use in children as young as 2 years of age).

Most important risks/adverse events:
Lactic acidosis and severe hepatomegaly with steatosis (boxed warning); severe acute exacerbations of hepatitis upon discontinuation of treatment (boxed warning); myopathy in conjunction with increases in creatine kinase (CK) values has been experienced by some patients, and patients should be advised to promptly report any unexplained muscle aches, pain, tenderness, or weakness.

Most common adverse events:
Upper respiratory tract infection (14%), fatigue and malaise (12%), abdominal pain (12%), nasopharyngitis (11%), headache (11%).

Usual dosage:

600 mg once a day; dosage interval should be increased in patients with impaired renal function.

Products:

Tablets – 600 mg; (an oral solution formulation [100 mg/5 mL] has been subsequently approved).

Comments:

Telbivudine is a thymidine nucleoside analogue that is phosphorylated to its active triphosphate form that inhibits HBV DNA polymerase (reverse transcriptase). It was compared with lamivudine in the pivotal study (GLOBE) that was the primary basis for its approval, and the one-year results of this study demonstrated a therapeutic response in approximately 75% of the patients treated with each of the two drugs. The second-year results of this study identified a higher therapeutic response rate in the patients treated with telbivudine. Telbivudine has not been directly compared with entecavir, a recently-marketed (2005) antiviral agent that has been effective in some patients with chronic HBV infection that has become resistant to lamivudine. There have not been well-controlled studies of telbivudine in patients with chronic HBV infections that have become resistant to any of the other antiviral agents.

Telbivudine appears more likely than the other agents for HBV infection to cause musculoskeletal effects (e.g., myopathy), and patients should be advised to promptly report any unexplained symptoms involving the musculature.

Temsirolimus (Torisel – Wyeth)
Antineoplastic Agent
2007

New Drug Comparison Rating (NDCR) = 4 (significant advantages)

Indication:
Administered via intravenous infusion for the treatment of advanced renal cell carcinoma.

Comparable drugs:
Sorafenib (Nexavar), sunitinib (Sutent). Additional comparable drugs, everolimus [Afinitor] and pazopanib [Votrient] were marketed in 2009.

Advantages:
- Unique mechanism of action for the treatment of cancer (inhibits the activity of mammalian target of rapamycin).
- May be effective in some patients who have not responded to other therapies.

Disadvantages:
- Administered intravenously (sorafenib and sunitinib are administered orally).
- More likely to cause hypersensitivity reactions.

Most important risks/adverse events:
Hypersensitivity reactions (an antihistamine should be administered prior to infusion of the drug); infection (risk is increased by immunosuppressive action); abnormal wound healing (use with caution in the perioperative period); interstitial lung disease; bowel perforation; renal failure; intracerebral hemorrhage; hyperglycemia; hyperlipemia; use of live vaccines should be avoided; may cause harm to a fetus and should not be used during pregnancy (precautions to avoid pregnancy should continue for 3 months following discontinuation of treatment); is a substrate for CYP3A4 and action may be increased by CYP3A4 inhibitors (e.g., clarithromycin [e.g., Biaxin]) and decreased by CYP3A4 inducers (e.g., rifampin [e.g., Rifadin]); St. John's wort should not be used concurrently.

Most common adverse events:
Asthenia (51%), rash (47%), mucositis (41%), nausea (37%), edema (35%), anorexia (32%), anemia (94%), hyperglycemia (89%), hyperlipemia (87%), hypertriglyceridemia (83%), elevated alkaline phosphatase (68%), elevated serum creatinine (57%), lymphopenia (53%), hypophosphatemia (49%), thrombocytopenia (40%).

Usual dosage:

Administered via intravenous infusion over 30-60 minutes; 25 mg once a week; treatment is continued until cancer worsens or there is unacceptable toxicity; if the concurrent use of a strong CYP3A4 inhibitor cannot be avoided, a reduction in dosage to 12.5 mg once a week should be considered; if the concurrent use of a strong CYP3A4 inducer cannot be avoided, an increase in dosage to 50 mg once a week should be considered; a 25 to 50 mg dose of diphenhydramine (e.g., Benadryl), or similar antihistamine, should be administered approximately 30 minutes before the start of each dose.

Product:

Vials – 25 mg/mL supplied in a kit that also includes the diluent; (should be stored in a refrigerator); diluent is a non-aqueous, ethanolic solution, and is injected into the vial containing the drug; volume of solution needed to provide the dose determined is withdrawn from the vial and injected into a 250 mL container of 0.9% Sodium Chloride Injection; to minimize patient exposure to the plasticizer DEHP (di-2-ethylhexyl phthalate) which may be leached from PVC infusion bags or sets (rate of extraction of DEHP is known to be increased by polysorbate 80 [included in the diluent]), the final temsirolimus dilution for infusion should be stored in bottles (glass, polypropylene) or plastic bags (polypropylene, polyolefin) and administered through polyethylene-lined administration sets.

Comments:

The principal active metabolite of temsirolimus is sirolimus (Rapamune), an immunosuppressant that was first marketed in 1999 for prophylaxis of organ rejection in patients receiving organ transplants. Sirolimus also is known as rapamycin, and it inhibits the activation of mammalian target of rapamycin (mTOR), a kinase that regulates cell proliferation, growth, and survival. Temsirolimus binds to an intracellular protein, and the protein-drug complex inhibits the activity of mTOR, resulting in reduced concentrations of cell growth factors and proliferation of certain cancer cell lines. Temsirolimus was compared with interferon alfa in clinical studies and the median overall survival was significantly longer in the patients receiving the new drug (10.9 months compared with 7.3 months). Additional drugs including everolimus and pazopanib have been marketed for the treatment of renal cell carcinoma, and bevacizumab (Avastin) has been approved for use in combination with interferon alfa.

Tetrabenazine (Xenazine – Lundbeck)
Agent for Chorea in Huntington's Disease
2008

New Drug Comparison Rating (NDCR) = 5 (important advance)

Indication:

Treatment of chorea associated with Huntington's disease.

Comparable drugs:

None.

Advantages:

• First drug to be demonstrated to be effective in treating chorea associated with Huntington's disease.

Disadvantages/Limitations:

• May increase risk of depression and suicidality.

Most important risks/adverse events:

Depression and suicidality (boxed warning; a Risk Evaluation and Mitigation Strategy [REMS] and Medication Guide have been developed); contraindicated in patients who are actively suicidal or in patients with untreated or inadequately treated depression; also contraindicated in patients with impaired hepatic function, and patients treated with a monoamine oxidase inhibitor or reserpine (at least 20 days should elapse following the discontinuation of reserpine before initiating treatment with tetrabenazine); hypotension; dysphagia; neuroleptic malignant syndrome; tardive dyskinesia; hyperprolactinemia; QT interval prolongation (should not be used concurrently with other drugs that prolong the QT interval or in patients with congenital long QT syndrome or a history of cardiac arrhythmias); activity is increased in patients who are poor metabolizers and in patients who are concurrently taking a strong CYP2D6 inhibitor (e.g., fluoxetine [e.g., Prozac], paroxetine [e.g., Paxil]).

Most common adverse events:

Sedation/somnolence (31%; patients should be cautioned about engaging in activities requiring mental alertness), fatigue (22%), insomnia (22%), depression (19%), akathisia (19%), anxiety (15%), nausea (13%), parkinsonism/bradykinesia (9%), balance difficulty (9%), irritability (9%).

205

Usual dosage:

Should be individualized; initial dosage – 12.5 mg once a day in the morning; after one week, the dosage should be increased to 12.5 mg twice a day; the dosage may be increased at weekly intervals by 12.5 mg; if a dosage of 37.5 mg or greater per day is needed, the drug should be administered in a three times a day regimen; maximum recommended daily dosage is 100 mg, and the maximum recommended single dose is 37.5 mg; patients who are considered likely to need a daily dosage above 50 mg should be genotyped for CYP2D6; in patients who are CYP2D6 poor metabolizers, or if treatment is to be initiated in patients already being treated with a stable dosage of a strong CYP2D6 inhibitor, the maximum recommended daily dosage is 50 mg and the maximum recommended single dose is 25 mg.

Products:

Tablets – 12.5 mg, 25 mg.

Comments:

Huntington's disease is a rare, inherited neurological disorder that is passed from parent to child through a gene mutation. The disease is associated with excessive activity of monoamines, primarily dopamine. Changes in personality or mood may be the earliest signs of the disease, followed by problems of memory and chorea (jerky, involuntary movements). Tetrabenazine is the first drug to be approved for the treatment of chorea associated with Huntington's disease. It reversibly inhibits the human vesicular monoamine transporter type 2 (VMAT2), resulting in depletion of monoamine stores. Its therapeutic benefit is thought to be primarily due to the depletion of dopamine. The effectiveness of tetrabenazine was demonstrated in a placebo-controlled study in which 50% of the treated patients attained the primary efficacy endpoint (improvement in the total chorea score) compared with 7% of those receiving placebo.

Although tetrabenazine is well tolerated by many patients, it may increase the risk of depression and suicidality and cause other serious adverse events. Appropriate precautions must be observed. Tetrabenazine is rapidly and extensively metabolized in the liver to alpha-dihydrotetrabenazine and beta-dihydrotetrabenazine that are pharmacologically active and the major circulating metabolites. These metabolites are further metabolized via the CYP2D6 pathway, and their activity is increased in poor metabolizers and in patients also taking a strong CYP2D6 inhibitor.

Tigecycline (Tygacil — Wyeth)
Antibiotic
2005

New Drug Comparison Rating (NDCR) = 4 (significant advantages)

Indications:

Administered via intravenous infusion for the treatment of complicated intra-abdominal infections and complicated skin and skin-structure infections caused by susceptible bacteria; may be initiated as empiric monotherapy before results of microbiological tests are known (subsequently approved for the treatment of community-acquired bacterial pneumonia).

Comparable drugs:

Tetracyclines (e.g., doxycycline [e.g., Vibramycin], minocycline [e.g., Minocin]), imipenem/cilastatin (Primaxin), combination antibiotic regimens (e.g., vancomycin and aztreonam).

Advantages:

- May be effective in the treatment of certain infections caused by bacteria that are not susceptible to other antibiotics.
- May be effective as monotherapy in certain infections that otherwise would need to be treated with combination antibiotic regimens.
- Cross-resistance with other antibiotics has not been observed.

Disadvantages:

- Associated with risks characteristic of the tetracyclines (e.g., use in children and during pregnancy) (compared with imipenem/cilastatin and combination antibiotic regimens).
- Oral bioavailability is limited and is not available in an oral dosage form (compared with doxycycline and minocycline).

Most important risks/adverse events:

May cause harm to the fetus if administered during pregnancy (Pregnancy Category D); risk of adverse events is increased in patients with severe hepatic impairment; although it is not indicated for use in patients under 18 years of age, permanent discoloration of the teeth may occur if used during the last half of pregnancy or childhood to the age of 8 years.

Most common adverse events:

Nausea (30%), vomiting (20%), diarrhea (13%), local reactions (9%), infection (8%), fever (7%), abdominal pain (7%).

Usual dosage:

100 mg initially via intravenous infusion over 30 to 60 minutes, followed by 50 mg every 12 hours; usual duration of treatment is 5 to 14 days; maintenance dosage should be reduced in patients with severe hepatic impairment.

Products:

Vials – 50 mg.

Comments:

Although sometimes designated as the first glycylcycline antibiotic, tigecycline is closely related structurally to minocycline and shares many of its actions and risks as well as those of the other tetracyclines. However, tigecycline is not apparently affected by the two major tetracycline resistance mechanisms, and cross-resistance between tigecycline and other antibiotics has not been observed. Tigecycline has a broad spectrum of action against numerous gram-positive and gram-negative aerobic and anaerobic bacteria, some of which (e.g., methicillin-resistant Staphylococcus aureus [MRSA]) have not demonstrated susceptibility to other tetracyclines. In the clinical studies, the clinical cure rates with its use were similar to those attained with imipenem/cilastatin or a combination of vancomycin and aztreonam. Its broad spectrum of action permits its use as empiric monotherapy before the results of microbiological tests are available, and as monotherapy in certain infections for which a combination of antibiotics has often been necessary.

Tigecycline is not extensively metabolized and its primary route of elimination is biliary excretion (approximately 60%) of unchanged drug.

Tipranavir (Aptivus — Boehringer Ingelheim)
Antiviral Agent
2005

New Drug Comparison Rating (NDCR) = 4 (significant advantages — see Comments))

Indication:
Coadministered with ritonavir and used with other antiretroviral agents for the treatment of HIV-1 infected adult patients with evidence of viral replication, who are highly treatment-experienced or have HIV-1 strains resistant to multiple protease inhibitors; (subsequently revised to include use in pediatric patients [2 to 18 years]).

Comparable drugs:
Amprenavir (Agenerase), atazanavir (Reyataz), fosamprenavir (Lexiva), indinavir (Crixivan), lopinavir/ritonavir (Kaletra), nelfinavir (Viracept), ritonavir (Norvir), saquinavir (Invirase); subsequent to the marketing of tipranavir, darunavir (Prezista) was also marketed.

Advantages:
- May be effective against HIV-1 strains that are resistant to most other protease inhibitors.

Disadvantages (identified at the time it was first marketed in 2005-see Comments):
- May be more likely to cause hepatic adverse events.
- Contains a sulfonamide moiety and may exhibit cross-sensitivity in sulfonamide-allergic patients (compared with atazanavir, indinavir, lopinavir/ritonavir, nelfinavir, ritonavir, and saquinavir).
- Administered twice a day (compared with atazanavir that is administered once a day).

Most important risks/adverse events:
Intracranial hemorrhage (boxed warning); clinical hepatitis and hepatic decompensation (boxed warning); contraindicated in patients with moderate or severe hepatic impairment; liver function tests should be frequently monitored; platelet aggregation inhibition; hyperglycemia; lipid elevations; risk of increased bleeding in patients with hemophilia; fat redistribution; immune reconstitution syndrome; rash; tipranavir/ritonavir inhibits the CYP3A and CYP2D6 metabolic pathways and increases the action of CYP3A and CYP2D6 substrates (contraindicated for concurrent use with midazolam [e.g., Versed], triazolam [e.g., Halcion], ergot-type products [e.g., dihydroergotamine], pimozide [e.g., Orap], amiodarone [e.g., Pacerone], bepridil [Vascor], flecainide [e.g., Tambocor], propafenone [Rythmol], and quinidine); concurrent use with lovastatin (e.g., Mevacor), simvastatin (e.g., Zocor), and fluticasone (Flovent) is not recommended; concurrent use may increase the activity of atorvastatin (Lipitor), fluoxetine (e.g., Prozac), paroxetine (e.g., Paxil), rifabutin (e.g., Mycobutin). phosphodiesterase type 5

inhibitors (e.g., sildenafil [Viagra]), and other CYP3A and CYP2D6 substrates (dosage for some agents may need to be reduced); may decrease the action of methadone and it may be necessary to increase the dosage of methadone; may decrease the action of ethinyl estradiol and women using estrogen-based oral contraceptives should use an alternative method of nonhormonal contraception; action may be reduced by use of rifampin (e.g., Rifadin) or St. John's wort and concurrent use with these agents is not recommended; interactions with other antiretroviral agents may occur and require dosage adjustment of one or more agents; structure contains a sulfonamide moiety and caution must be exercised in patients with a history of sulfonamide allergy.

Most common adverse events:

ALT and/or AST elevations (18%), rash (12%), diarrhea (11%).

Usual dosage:

Adults - 500 mg coadministered with 200 mg of ritonavir twice a day; pediatric patients (2 to 18 years) – 14 mg/kg with 6 mg/kg ritonavir (or 375 mg/m^2 with 150 mg/m^2 ritonavir) a day.

Product:

Capsules – 250 mg (should be stored in a refrigerator); oral solution – 100 mg/mL.

Comments:

Unlike the previously marketed HIV protease inhibitors that are large peptides, tipranavir does not have a peptide structure. It has demonstrated activity against HIV strains that are resistant to other protease inhibitors. Tipranavir must be coadministered with ritonavir and its use should be reserved for treatment-experienced patients who show evidence of resistance to other protease inhibitors. Its NDCR of 4 was determined at the time of its initial marketing, and the subsequent approval of darunavir (Prezista) reduces its importance.

Tolvaptan (Samsca – Otsuka)
Agent for Hyponatremia
2009

New Drug Comparison Rating (NDCR) = 4 (significant advantages)

Indication:

For the treatment of clinically significant hypervolemic and euvolemic hyponatremia (serum sodium less than 125 mEq/L or less marked hyponatremia that is symptomatic and has resisted correction with fluid restriction), including patients with heart failure, cirrhosis, and Syndrome of Inappropriate Antidiuretic Hormone (SIADH).

Comparable drug:

Conivaptan (Vaprisol).

Advantages:

- Is administered orally (whereas conivaptan is administered intravenously).
- Duration of use is not restricted (treatment with conivaptan should not be continued for longer than 4 days) and maintenance treatment does not require hospitalization.

Disadvantages:

- Should not be used to raise serum sodium urgently to prevent or to treat serious neurologic symptoms.

Most important risks/adverse events:

Contraindicated in patients with an urgent need to raise sodium acutely, patients who are unable to sense or appropriately respond to thirst, patients with hypovolemic hyponatremia, and patients who are anuric; action may be significantly increased by the concurrent use of CYP3A inhibitors (concurrent use with a strong CYP3A inhibitor [e.g., clarithromycin] is contraindicated, and the use of moderate CYP3A inhibitors [e.g., diltiazem, grapefruit juice] should be avoided); too rapid correction of hyponatremia (e.g., more than 12 mEq/L/24 hours) must be avoided (boxed warning) as osmotic demyelination and serious complications may result; treatment should be initiated and re-initiated in a hospital (boxed warning); gastrointestinal bleeding in patients with cirrhosis; dehydration and hypovolemia (as a consequence of copious aquaresis); hyperkalemia (should be monitored in patients with a serum potassium greater than 5 mEq/L and in patients receiving other drugs known to increase serum potassium concentrations); action may be reduced by the concurrent use of CYP3A inducers (e.g., rifampin), and increased by P-glycoprotein inhibitors (e.g., cyclosporine).

Most common adverse events:

Thirst (16%), dry mouth (13%), pollakiuria (extraordinary urinary frequency) or polyuria (11%), asthenia (9%), constipation (7%), hyperglycemia (6%).

Usual dosage:

Treatment should be initiated and re-initiated in a hospital; initial dosage is 15 mg once a day; dosage may be increased to 30 mg once a day, after at least 24 hours, to a maximum of 60 mg once a day as needed; patients should be advised that they can continue ingestion of fluid in response to thirst; when treatment is discontinued, patients should be advised to resume fluid restriction.

Products:

Tablets – 15 mg, 30 mg.

Comments:

Patients with hyponatremia may be asymptomatic but, as sodium concentrations decrease, neurologic symptoms (e.g., headache, confusion, seizures) may result. Dilutional hyponatremia is the most common form. The hormone arginine vasopressin (AVP), also known as antidiuretic hormone, regulates water loss from the body by altering water permeability of the renal collecting ducts, primarily by acting at vasopressin V2 receptors. Hypervolemic hyponatremia is often associated with underlying conditions such as congestive heart failure and cirrhosis of the liver, whereas euvolemic hyponatremia is often associated with the syndrome of inappropriate antidiuretic hormone. Conivaptan is an AVP antagonist that acts primarily at V2 receptors. It is administered intravenously in hospitalized patients for a period of treatment that should not exceed 4 days. Tolvaptan is a selective vasopressin V2 receptor antagonist that is administered orally. Its effectiveness was demonstrated in studies in which patients were treated for 30 days with either tolvaptan or placebo. Serum sodium concentrations increased to a significantly greater degree in tolvaptan-treated patients as early as 8 hours after the first dose.

Too rapid correction of hyponatremia is the most important risk with the use of tolvaptan.

Ustekinumab (Stelara – Centocor Ortho Biotech)
Agent for Psoriasis
2009

New Drug Comparison Rating (NDCR) = 4 (significant advantages)

Indication:
Administered subcutaneously for the treatment of adult patients with moderate to severe plaque psoriasis who are candidates for phototherapy or systemic therapy.

Comparable drug:
Etanercept (Enbrel).

Advantages:
- Unique mechanism of action (interleukin-12 and -23 antagonist).
- More effective than etanercept in a comparative study.
- Less frequent administration (every 12 weeks for maintenance treatment compared with once weekly maintenance treatment with etanercept).
- May be associated with a lesser risk of infection (compared with a boxed warning regarding this risk in the labeling for etanercept).

Disadvantages:
- Labeled indications are more limited (etanercept also has labeled indications for rheumatoid arthritis, polyarticular juvenile idiopathic arthritis, ankylosing spondylitis, and psoriatic arthritis).
- Should only be administered by a healthcare provider (whereas etanercept may be self-administered).

Most important risks/adverse events:
Risk of infections (should not be used in patients with clinically important active infections; patients should be evaluated for tuberculosis prior to initiating treatment); risk of malignancies (as a result of immunosuppressant action); reversible posterior leukoencephalopathy syndrome (one case report in clinical studies); patients should not receive live vaccines during period of treatment (all immunizations appropriate for age should be administered prior to initiating therapy).

Most common adverse events:
Nasopharyngitis (7%), headache (5%), upper respiratory tract infection (4%), fatigue (3%).

Usual dosage:

Administered subcutaneously; in patients weighing 100 kg or less, the recommended dosage is 45 mg initially and 4 weeks later, followed by 45 mg every 12 weeks; in patients weighing more than 100 kg, the recommended dosage is 90 mg initially and 4 weeks later, followed by 90 mg every 12 weeks.

Products:

Single-use vials – 45 mg/0.5 mL, 90 mg/1 mL (should be stored in a refrigerator).

Comments:

Advances in the treatment of moderate to severe plaque psoriasis have included the use of tumor necrosis factor (TNF) inhibitors (etanercept, adalimumab [Humira], infliximab [Remicade]), and alefacept (Amevive) that interferes with T-cell activation. Interleukin-12 (IL-12) and interleukin-23 (IL-23) are naturally-occurring proteins that are also thought to have a role in the occurrence and worsening of psoriasis. Ustekinumab is a human monoclonal antibody that is the first drug to selectively target and bind these cytokines. In two placebo-controlled clinical studies, approximately 70% of patients treated with the new drug achieved at least a 75% reduction in psoriasis after two doses, compared with less than 5% of those receiving placebo. Patients were evaluated through one year and approximately 90% of those having at least a 75% reduction in psoriasis maintained this response through one year of treatment. In a study in which ustekinumab was compared with etanercept, 68% and 74% of patients treated with 45 mg and 90 mg dosages of ustekinumab, respectively, experienced at least a 75% reduction in psoriasis, compared with 57% of the patients treated with etanercept.

Ustekinumab has a long duration of action and following the first two doses at weeks 0 and 4, subsequent doses are administered every 12 weeks. In the maintenance treatment of plaque psoriasis, etanercept is administered once a week, adalimumab once every 2 weeks, infliximab (intravenously) once every 8 weeks, and alefacept (intramuscularly) once a week.

Varenicline tartrate (Chantix – Pfizer)
Agent for Smoking Cessation
2006

New Drug Comparison Rating (NDCR) = 5 (important advance)

Indication:

As an aid in smoking cessation treatment.

Comparable drugs:

Bupropion sustained-release (e.g., Zyban).

Advantages:

- Has a unique mechanism of action.
- Greater effectiveness has been demonstrated in comparative studies.
- Not likely to cause serious adverse events (postmarketing experience suggests a potential for suicidal thoughts and erratic behavior).
- Not likely to interact with other drugs.

Disadvantages:

- More likely to cause nausea.
- Experience is more limited.
- Recommended dosage guidelines include one more titration step.

Most important risks/adverse events:

Is excreted unchanged in the urine and dosage should be reduced in patients with severe renal impairment; (postmarketing experience has included reports of suicidal thoughts and erratic behavior, and a boxed warning has been added to the labeling; reports of drowsiness warrant caution when driving or engaging in other potentially hazardous activities).

Most common adverse events:

Nausea (30%), insomnia (18%), abnormal dreams (13%), constipation (8%), flatulence (6%), vomiting (5%).

Usual dosage:

Smoker should determine a date to stop smoking and varenicline treatment should be initiated one week before this date; should be administered after eating and with a full glass of water; initial dosage is 0.5 mg once a day on days 1-3, followed by 0.5 mg twice a day in the morning and evening on days 4-7, followed by 1 mg twice a day from day 8

215

until the end of treatment; a course of treatment should continue for 12 weeks; for patients who have stopped smoking at the end of 12 weeks, an additional 12-week course of treatment is recommended to increase the likelihood of long-term abstinence.

Products:

0.5 mg, 1 mg, supplied in packs containing both potencies to facilitate dosage titration.

Comments:

Pharmacologic options to help individuals stop smoking have included the nicotine replacement therapy (NRT) formulations and bupropion sustained-release. Varenicline is a partial agonist selective for $alpha_4beta_2$ nicotinic acetylcholine receptor subtypes. It binds with high affinity to these receptors and its agonist action is thought to reduce the craving to smoke as well as the withdrawal symptoms from nicotine. By occupying these receptor sites, varenicline prevents the binding of nicotine if the individual smokes while receiving treatment, thereby reducing the satisfaction associated with smoking.

In studies in which varenicline was compared with bupropion sustained-release, abstinence from smoking was evaluated during weeks 9-12 of the studies. Varenicline was determined to be effective in 44% of the participants, compared with 30% of those receiving bupropion and 17% of those receiving placebo. Continuing studies in which varenicline was compared with placebo demonstrated higher abstinence rates after 24 weeks of treatment and following a 28-week post-treatment period.

The use of bupropion is associated with risks such as seizures, suicidality, and a potential for interactions with numerous other medications. There were no reports of serious adverse events with varenicline in clinical trials. However, in the postmarketing experience, there have been reports of suicidal thoughts, erratic behavior, and drowsiness. None of the NRT formulations provides the optimum balance of onset of action and duration of action and, even though the use of NRT is much safer than continuing to smoke, it represents a continuing source of the agent (nicotine) to which the individual is addicted.

Vigabatrin (Sabril – Lundbeck)
Antiepileptic Drug
2009

New Drug Comparison Rating (NDCR) = 5 (important advance)

Indications:
Monotherapy for pediatric patients (1 month to 2 years of age) with infantile spasms for whom the potential benefits outweigh the potential risk of vision loss; also indicated as adjunctive therapy for adult patients with refractory complex partial seizures who have inadequately responded to several alternative treatments and for whom the potential benefits outweigh the risk of vision loss (is not indicated as a first-line agent for complex partial seizures).

Comparable drugs:
None.

Advantages:
- First drug to be approved for the treatment of infantile spasms.
- May be effective in some patients with complex partial seizures who are refractory to other therapies.

Disadvantages/Limitations:
- Risk of vision loss.
- May be less effective than certain agents that are used "off-label" for the treatment of infantile spasms.

Most important risks/adverse events:
May cause permanent vision loss (boxed warning; progressive loss of peripheral vision with potential decrease in visual acuity; vision should be assessed at baseline and at least every 3 months during therapy; vision testing is also required about 3-6 months following discontinuation of therapy); abnormal magnetic resonance imaging (MRI) abnormalities (involving the thalamus, basal ganglia, brain stem, and cerebellum in some infants with infantile spasms); neurotoxicity (observed in animals and characterized by fluid accumulation and separation of the outer layers of myelin [intramyelinic edema]); suicidal ideation and behavior (adult patients should be monitored for the emergence or worsening of depression, suicidal thoughts, and/or unusual changes in mood or behavior); peripheral neuropathy; anemia; somnolence and fatigue; edema, weight gain; may reduce plasma concentrations of phenytoin.

Most common adverse events:
In patients with infantile spasms – somnolence (45%), bronchitis (30%), ear infection (10%), acute otitis media (10%); when used in combination with other antiepileptic drugs – headache (18%), somnolence (17%), fatigue (16%), dizziness (15%), convulsion (11%), nasopharyngitis (10%), weight gain (10%), upper respiratory tract infection (10%), visual field defect (9%), depression (8%), nystagmus (7%), blurred vision (6%), diplopia (6%).

Usual dosage:

Infantile spasms – 50 mg/kg/day in two divided doses initially; can be titrated by 25-50 mg/kg/day increments every 3 days up to a maximum of 150 mg/kg/day; refractory complex partial seizures – 500 mg twice a day initially; may be increased in 500 mg increments at weekly intervals to the recommended dosage of 1500 mg twice a day; dosage should be reduced in patients with renal impairment; if treatment is to be discontinued, dosage should be gradually reduced.

Products:

Tablets – 500 mg; powder for oral solution – 500 mg packet; powder should be placed in an empty cup and dissolved in 10 mL of cold or room temperature water per packet using the 10 mL oral syringe supplied with the medication (concentration of the final solution is 50 mg/mL).

Comments:

Infantile spasms usually appear in the first year of life and primarily consist of a sudden bending forward of the body with stiffening of the arms and legs. Spasms tend to occur upon awakening or after feeding, and often occur in clusters of up to 100 spasms. Infants may experience dozens of clusters and several hundred spasms per day. Agents such as prednisolone and adrenocorticotropic hormone (ACTH) have been used "off-label" in the treatment of infantile spasms but vigabatrin is the first drug to be approved for the treatment of this condition. Its specific mechanism of action is not known but is thought to result from its action as an irreversible inhibitor of gamma-aminobutyric acid transaminase (GABA-T), the enzyme responsible for the metabolism of the inhibitory neurotransmitter GABA. This action results in increased concentrations of GABA in the central nervous system.

The effectiveness of vigabatrin in the treatment of infantile spasms was demonstrated in a study in which infants received either a low dosage or high dosage of the drug. The primary efficacy endpoint was the proportion of patients who were spasm-free for 7 consecutive days. Sixteen percent of the patients in the high-dose group achieved spasm freedom compared with 7% of those in the low-dose group. In limited comparative studies, vigabatrin has been considered less effective than ACTH in the treatment of infantile spasms. This is not a labeled indication for ACTH although a supplemental new drug application has been submitted seeking approval for this indication.

Vigabatrin is not a first-line treatment for complex partial seizures and should only be considered for use in patients whose condition is refractory to several other antiepileptic drugs.

Vigabatrin may cause permanent vision loss in infants, children, and adults. It causes bilateral concentric visual field constriction in 30% or more of patients that ranges in severity from mild to severe, including tunnel vision, and can result in disability. In some patients, the drug may also damage the central retina and decrease visual acuity. The onset of vision loss is unpredictable and can occur at any time during treatment. Because of the risk of vision loss, vigabatrin should be withdrawn from patients with infantile spasms who fail to show substantial clinical benefit within 2 to 4 weeks of initiation of treatment. The drug is available only through a restricted distribution program (1-888-45-SHARE). Only prescribers and pharmacies who are registered in this program may prescribe and distribute vigabatrin for patients who meet the conditions of and are enrolled in the program.

Vorinostat (Zolinza – Merck)
Antineoplastic Agent
2006

New Drug Comparison Rating (NDCR) = 4 (significant advantages)

Indication:
Treatment of cutaneous manifestations in patients with cutaneous T-cell lymphoma who have progressive, persistent or recurrent disease on or following two systemic therapies.

Comparable drugs:
Bexarotene (Targretin).

Advantages:
- Has a unique mechanism of action (inhibits histone deacetylases).
- May be effective in some patients with cutaneous T-cell lymphoma who have not responded adequately to or have not tolerated other therapies.
- Less likely to cause lipid abnormalities and pancreatitis.

Disadvantages:
- Labeled indication is more limited (bexarotene is indicated in patients who are refractory to at least one prior systemic therapy).
- Risk of pulmonary embolism and deep vein thrombosis.
- May cause QT interval prolongation.
- May cause hyperglycemia.

Most important risks/adverse events:
Pulmonary embolism and deep vein thrombosis; thrombocytopenia and anemia (blood cell counts, platelet counts, and chemistry tests including electrolytes, glucose, and serum creatinine should be monitored every 2 weeks during the first 2 months of therapy and at least monthly thereafter); QT interval prolongation (electrocardiograms and electrolytes should be monitored); hyperglycemia; gastrointestinal adverse events (e.g., bleeding, vomiting, diarrhea, dehydration [patients should be advised to drink at least eight 8-ounce glasses of liquid per day]); may cause harm to a fetus and should not be used during pregnancy; concurrent use with another histone deacetylase inhibitor (e.g., valproic acid) has been associated with severe thrombocytopenia and gastrointestinal bleeding); concurrent use with warfarin (e.g., Coumadin) has resulted in prolongation of prothrombin time and the International Normalized Ratio (INR).

Most common adverse events:
Fatigue (52%), diarrhea (52%), nausea (41%), dysgeusia (28%), thrombocytopenia (26%), anorexia (24%), weight loss (32%), muscle spasms (20%).

Usual dosage:

400 mg once a day with food.

Products:

Capsules – 100 mg.

Comments:

Cutaneous T-cell lymphoma (CTCL) is a general term for a group of non-Hodgkin's lymphomas in which malignant T cells typically manifest initially in the skin. Skin lesions are often pruritic and painful, and may become ulcerative and necrotic. Systemic involvement of the lymph nodes, spleen, liver, or other viscera can occur with time. In the earliest stages of the disorder, emollients, antipruritics, and topical corticosteroids are used to control symptoms. As the condition worsens, topical treatments such as psoralens and ultraviolet radiation have been used, as have chemotherapies such as bexarotene.

Vorinostat has a mechanism of action that is unique among the antineoplastic agents. It inhibits the activity of histone deacetylases (HDACs), enzymes that catalyze the removal of acetyl groups from the lysine residues of proteins, including histones and transcription factors. In some cancer cells, there is an overexpression of HDACs and the inhibition of HDAC activity by vorinostat confers a beneficial response in some patients with CTCL. In the largest clinical trial, the overall response rate was 30% and the median time to response 55 days, although it took up to 6 months for some patients to achieve an objective response. The median duration of response was estimated to be more than 6 months.

Ziconotide (Prialt – Elan)
Analgesic
2005

New Drug Comparison Rating (NDCR) = 4 (significant advantages)

Indication:
Administered via intrathecal injection for the management of severe chronic pain in patients for whom intrathecal therapy is warranted, and who are intolerant of or refractory to other treatment, such as systemic analgesics, adjunctive therapies, or intrathecal morphine.

Comparable drugs:
Morphine.

Advantages:
- May be effective in relieving pain in patients who are refractory to or intolerant of other agents.
- Unique mechanism of action (binds to N-type calcium channels).
- Not addictive.

Disadvantages:
- May cause severe psychiatric symptoms and neurologic impairment.
- Must be administered by the intrathecal route of administration.

Most important risks/adverse events:
Psychiatric symptoms and neurologic impairment (boxed warning; contraindicated in patients with a history of psychosis); musculoskeletal adverse events (serum creatine kinase [CK] concentrations should be monitored); risk of meningitis that may result from inadvertent contamination of the microinfusion device.

Most common adverse events:
Dizziness (47%), nausea (41%), confusion (33%), memory impairment (22%), asthenia (22%), somnolence (22%), headache (15%), speech disorder (14%), hallucinations (12%), aphasia (12%), CK elevations (40%).

Usual dosage:
Administered via intrathecal infusion; initial dosage – 2.4 mcg/day (0.1 mcg/hour)—is then titrated upward to patient response by up to 2.4 mcg/day at intervals of no more than 2 to 3 times per week, up to a recommended maximum dosage of 19.2 mcg/day by day 21; intended for use in the Medtronic SynchroMed EL or SynchroMed II infusion systems, or Deltec Cadd-Micro external microinfusion device and catheter.

Products:

Vials – 100 mcg/mL (1 mL, 2 mL, 5 mL vials [should be diluted]); vials – 25 mcg/mL (20 mL [may be used undiluted]).

Comments:

Ziconotide is a synthetic 25-amino acid peptide that is equivalent to a naturally occurring conopeptide found in the venom of a marine snail. It is a potent analgesic that binds to N-type calcium channels located on the primary nociceptive afferent nerves in the superficial layers of the dorsal horn in the spinal cord, possibly blocking them on the nerves that transmit pain signals to the brain. It does not bind to opiate receptors, its actions are not blocked by opiate antagonists, and it does not cause addiction.

Ziconotide is administered via intrathecal infusion using a programmable implanted microinfusion device or an external microinfusion device and catheter. Clinical studies of its use were conducted primarily in patients whose pain was refractory to intrathecal therapy (e.g., morphine). Many patients experience psychiatric, neurologic, and/or gastrointestinal adverse events; serious adverse events occur less frequently when the dosage is slowly titrated over 21 days than when a more rapid titration schedule is used.

Therapeutic Classification and/or Indication Index

The year in which the new drug was first marketed is noted following the name of the drug. When more than one new drug is listed for a particular therapeutic class and/or indication, they are listed in chronological order based on the year in which they were first marketed.

Therapeutic class/Indication   **Page**

Therapeutic class/Indication   Page

Therapeutic class/Indication	Page

Therapeutic class/Indication	Page

Therapeutic class/Indication	Page

Generic Name/Trade Name Index

Generic names are in **bold type** and trade names are in regular type and indented. The New Drug Comparison Ratings (NDCR) are also identified.

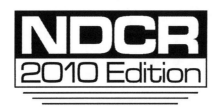

Visit our website at:
www.NewDrugsNDCR.com

4849829R0

Made in the USA
Charleston, SC
25 March 2010